The 5-Ingredient Mediterranean Dash Diet Cookbook

2000 Days of Delicious and Low-Sodium Recipes Ready in Less Than 25 Minutes Perfect to Lower Blood Pressure, Improve Heart Health and Lose Weight

Jane Manson

Table of Contents

Thank you so much for purchasing my book! I'm thrilled to have you as part of my reading family.

If you could take a moment to scan the QR code below and leave your honest review on Amazon, I would be deeply grateful.

If you are reading the ebook version, please click on this link:

https://www.amazon.com/review/create-review?&ASIN=B0DJC2P7W5

Your feedback is incredibly important to me—it helps me grow as a writer and makes our community stronger. I genuinely love hearing from you and value your thoughts immensely!

Introduction

Welcome to the 5-Ingredient Mediterranean DASH Diet Cookbook, a comprehensive guide designed to revolutionize your approach to eating and health. This book is your ally in achieving optimal health outcomes through a unique fusion of the Mediterranean and DASH diets, both celebrated for their benefits in lowering blood pressure, improving heart health, and aiding in weight management. For those beginning their journey towards a healthier lifestyle, this cookbook simplifies the process, offering easy-to-follow recipes that require no more than five ingredients each. The focus is on whole foods, rich in nutrients, that are both accessible and budget-friendly, making healthy eating an achievable goal for busy individuals.

To utilize this cookbook for optimal results, start by familiarizing yourself with the foundational principles of the Mediterranean and DASH diets outlined in the initial chapters. Understanding the science behind these diets and their proven benefits will empower you to make informed choices about your nutrition. The recipes are structured to minimize preparation time without compromising on taste or nutritional value, perfect for those with a demanding schedule. Each recipe is accompanied by a brief explanation of how it fits within the dietary guidelines, ensuring you can mix and match dishes to cater to your personal health goals.

Incorporating these meals into your daily routine is made simpler with the inclusion of a weekly shopping list, highlighting budget-friendly ingredients that form the basis of the recipes within this book. Additionally, learning to read and understand food labels is crucial in making healthier choices, a skill that this cookbook aims to impart through practical advice.

By embracing the principles and recipes in this cookbook, you embark on a journey towards improved well-being. The 5-Ingredient Mediterranean DASH Diet Cookbook is not just a collection of recipes; it's a lifestyle guide that promises to enhance your health without sacrificing flavor or convenience.

Chapter 1: Getting Started

The fusion of the Mediterranean and DASH diets creates a powerful dietary strategy designed to combat hypertension, improve heart health, and foster weight management. The Mediterranean diet, rich in fruits, vegetables, whole grains, and healthy fats, primarily olive oil, emphasizes the consumption of nutrient-dense, whole foods. This diet has been celebrated for its cardiovascular benefits and its role in promoting longevity and reducing the risk of chronic diseases. The DASH (Dietary Approaches to Stop Hypertension) diet, on the other hand, focuses on reducing sodium intake and increasing consumption of foods rich in potassium, calcium, and magnesium to lower blood pressure. By combining these two diets, individuals can leverage the health benefits of both, enjoying a flavorful and diverse array of foods that not only contribute to a healthier lifestyle but also support sustainable weight loss and energy levels.

To embark on this dietary journey, beginners should start with understanding the fundamental principles of both diets. Emphasizing the consumption of vegetables, fruits, whole grains, and lean proteins, while minimizing the intake of processed foods, sweets, and high-sodium products, is key. Transitioning to this dietary pattern may require a shift in cooking methods and meal planning but promises significant health benefits. Incorporating low-sodium cooking techniques and utilizing herbs and spices can enhance flavor without the need for excess salt, making meals both delicious and heart-healthy.

As individuals navigate this dietary transition, it's important to focus on gradual changes, such as introducing more vegetables into meals, opting for whole grains, and choosing lean protein sources. This approach not only makes the dietary shift more manageable but also ensures that the changes are sustainable in the long term. By adopting the principles of the Mediterranean DASH diet, individuals can look forward to not only lowering their blood pressure and improving their heart health but also achieving their weight loss goals and enhancing their overall well-being.

The Science Behind Mediterranean and DASH Diets

The Mediterranean and DASH diets, both acclaimed for their health benefits, are grounded in extensive scientific research. These diets share a common foundation: they emphasize the consumption of whole foods, fruits, vegetables, whole grains, lean proteins, and healthy fats, while limiting processed foods, red meats, and high-sodium items. The science behind these diets provides compelling evidence for their effectiveness in improving cardiovascular health, managing weight, and reducing the risk of chronic diseases.

The Mediterranean diet is inspired by the traditional eating habits of countries bordering the Mediterranean Sea. It is rich in fruits, vegetables, whole grains, olive oil, and fish, providing a high intake of dietary fiber, antioxidants, and mono- and polyunsaturated fats. Numerous studies have highlighted its benefits, including a landmark study published in the New England

Journal of Medicine, which demonstrated that the Mediterranean diet significantly reduced the risk of cardiovascular diseases, including heart attacks and strokes, among high-risk individuals. This diet's effectiveness is attributed to its ability to improve cholesterol levels, lower blood pressure, and reduce inflammation, all of which are risk factors for heart disease and stroke.

The DASH diet, short for Dietary Approaches to Stop Hypertension, was developed to lower blood pressure without medication. It focuses on eating foods rich in potassium, calcium, and magnesium—nutrients that help control blood pressure—and limiting foods high in sodium, saturated fat, and added sugars. Clinical trials, such as those conducted by the National Institutes of Health (NIH), have shown that the DASH diet can significantly lower systolic and diastolic blood pressure in individuals with hypertension. Furthermore, when combined with sodium reduction, the DASH diet's effects on blood pressure are even more pronounced, making it a powerful dietary strategy for hypertension management.

Both diets also play a significant role in weight management. The high fiber content in both diets contributes to satiety, helping individuals feel full longer and reducing overall calorie intake. While the primary focus of these diets is not weight loss, many people find that following these dietary patterns helps them achieve and maintain a healthy weight due to the emphasis on nutrient-dense, lower-calorie foods.

In combining the Mediterranean and DASH diets, individuals can harness the benefits of both: the heart-healthy fats and diverse plant-based foods of the Mediterranean diet, along with the blood pressure-lowering effects of the DASH diet's nutrient-rich, low-sodium approach. This synergistic combination offers a comprehensive dietary strategy that not only addresses specific health issues like hypertension and heart disease but also promotes overall well-being.

The scientific evidence supporting these diets underscores the importance of dietary patterns in managing health and preventing disease. By focusing on whole foods and balanced nutrition, the Mediterranean and DASH diets offer a sustainable approach to eating that can lead to long-term health benefits. As more research emerges, the scientific community continues to endorse these diets as effective tools for improving health outcomes, validating their significance in the field of nutritional science.

Benefits of Combining the Two Diets

The fusion of the Mediterranean and DASH diets creates a powerful synergy that amplifies the health benefits of each diet individually. This combination leverages the rich, diverse flavors of the Mediterranean diet with the structured, nutrient-focused approach of the DASH diet to offer a comprehensive lifestyle that supports heart health, blood pressure management, weight control, and overall well-being. The Mediterranean diet, celebrated for its use of whole grains, lean proteins, healthy fats, and an abundance of fruits and vegetables, aligns perfectly with the DASH diet's emphasis on low sodium and nutrient-rich foods to combat hypertension.

Together, they form a dietary pattern that is not only sustainable and enjoyable but also backed by scientific evidence for its health benefits.

One of the primary benefits of combining these two diets is the enhanced effect on cardiovascular health. Both diets independently have been shown to reduce the risk of heart disease, but when combined, they offer a more potent defense against hypertension and other cardiovascular risk factors. The Mediterranean diet's high intake of antioxidants and healthy fats, such as omega-3 fatty acids found in fish, has been linked to lower levels of LDL (bad) cholesterol and higher levels of HDL (good) cholesterol. Meanwhile, the DASH diet's focus on reducing sodium intake and increasing potassium-rich foods further aids in lowering blood pressure. Together, these dietary strategies can significantly reduce the risk of stroke and heart attack.

Weight management is another key benefit of merging the Mediterranean and DASH diets. Both diets emphasize whole foods over processed options and encourage eating a variety of nutrient-dense foods. This approach naturally leads to a reduction in calorie intake without the need for strict calorie counting, making it easier to achieve and maintain a healthy weight. The high fiber content from fruits, vegetables, and whole grains in both diets also promotes satiety, reducing the likelihood of overeating and supporting sustainable weight loss.

Furthermore, the combined diet offers a diverse palette of flavors and ingredients, making it easier to stick to in the long term compared to more restrictive diets. This diversity not only prevents dietary boredom but also ensures a wide range of vitamins, minerals, and antioxidants are consumed, supporting overall health. The inclusion of nuts, seeds, legumes, and lean proteins provides a balanced intake of essential nutrients, such as magnesium, calcium, and potassium, which are key components of the DASH diet for blood pressure management.

Another significant benefit is the potential for improved mental health and cognitive function. The Mediterranean diet, in particular, has been associated with a lower risk of cognitive decline and Alzheimer's disease. When combined with the DASH diet, which promotes overall health and well-being, it's plausible to suggest a synergistic effect that further supports brain health.

In conclusion, the combination of the Mediterranean and DASH diets offers a holistic approach to health that goes beyond the benefits of each diet alone. By focusing on nutrient-dense, flavorful foods that promote satiety and heart health, this fusion diet presents a viable, enjoyable path to long-term health and wellness, making it an ideal choice for anyone looking to improve their dietary habits and overall health.

Tips for Low-Sodium Cooking Without Sacrificing Flavor

Achieving flavorful meals without relying heavily on salt requires a blend of creativity and understanding of how various ingredients interact to enhance taste. The key to low-sodium cooking lies in leveraging the natural flavors of foods and employing techniques and seasonings that bring out their essence without the need for excess salt. One fundamental approach is the use of herbs and spices which can transform a simple dish into a complex, aromatic experience. Fresh herbs like basil, cilantro, rosemary, and thyme offer a burst of flavor that can elevate any meal. Similarly, spices such as cumin, paprika, turmeric, and cinnamon add depth and warmth, allowing for a reduction in salt without compromising taste.

Acidity is another powerful element in the culinary arsenal against blandness. The addition of lemon juice, lime, or vinegar can brighten dishes, giving them a fresh edge that salt might otherwise provide. These acidic components can be particularly effective in salads, seafood, and even in some desserts, offering a counterbalance to the richness of the other ingredients.

Another technique involves the use of umami-rich ingredients which impart a savory depth of flavor that can make dishes more satisfying. Foods like tomatoes, mushrooms, seaweed, and aged cheeses contain natural glutamates that enhance the taste experience similar to how salt does but without the negative health impacts associated with high sodium intake. Incorporating these ingredients into meals can significantly boost flavor profiles.

Roasting and caramelizing vegetables is a method that naturally intensifies the sweetness and flavor of the produce, reducing the need for added salt. This process involves cooking vegetables at a high temperature until they begin to brown and caramelize, releasing their natural sugars. Onions, carrots, and bell peppers are particularly well-suited to this technique and can serve as a flavorful base for a variety of dishes.

Lastly, building layers of flavor through the use of stocks and broths can add complexity to meals. Opting for low-sodium or homemade versions allows for control over the salt content while still infusing dishes with rich, savory notes. Whether used as a base for soups and stews or for cooking grains like rice or quinoa, these liquids contribute moisture and flavor, making them an invaluable tool in low-sodium cooking.

By focusing on these strategies, it's possible to create dishes that are both nutritious and full of taste, proving that a low-sodium diet does not have to be a bland one. Through the thoughtful combination of herbs, spices, acidity, umami, and careful cooking techniques, meals can be both healthful and delicious, aligning with the goals of the Mediterranean DASH diet to support heart health and overall well-being without sacrificing enjoyment of food.

Chapter 2: Diets and Their Benefits

The Mediterranean and DASH diets, both celebrated for their cardiovascular benefits, share a remarkable synergy that can significantly enhance one's health. At the core of these diets lies a focus on whole foods, emphasizing fruits, vegetables, whole grains, and lean proteins, while minimizing the intake of processed foods, red meats, and high-sodium items. This alignment between the two diets not only simplifies adherence for individuals seeking to improve their heart health and lower blood pressure but also amplifies the potential health benefits through a combined dietary approach.

The Mediterranean diet, with its rich history rooted in the eating habits of countries bordering the Mediterranean Sea, is renowned for its use of olive oil, a healthy fat that has been linked to reducing the risk of heart disease. The diet also encourages the consumption of nuts, seeds, and fish, which are high in omega-3 fatty acids, known for their anti-inflammatory properties and role in heart health. On the other hand, the DASH diet, which stands for Dietary Approaches to Stop Hypertension, is a scientifically formulated eating plan specifically designed to combat high blood pressure. It emphasizes the importance of potassium, calcium, and magnesium while recommending a reduced intake of sodium, sweets, and beverages containing sugar.

The convergence of these diets presents a powerful tool for individuals aiming to not only lower their blood pressure but also to lose weight and improve overall heart health. The reduction of sodium intake, a cornerstone of the DASH diet, when combined with the Mediterranean diet's focus on healthy fats and lean proteins, can lead to a more balanced and heart-healthy lifestyle. Furthermore, both diets advocate for moderate physical activity, which complements the dietary changes and contributes to the overall cardiovascular benefits.

The benefits of merging these two diets extend beyond heart health. Weight loss, improved metabolic health, and a lower risk of certain types of cancer have also been associated with adherence to these dietary patterns. The emphasis on whole foods and the diversity of nutrients provided by the Mediterranean-DASH diet fusion can also lead to improved energy levels, better digestion, and a more satisfying and sustainable eating plan.

For individuals concerned about the long-term implications of hypertension, diabetes, and heart disease, adopting a combined Mediterranean-DASH diet offers a practical and effective strategy to mitigate these risks. The approachable nature of these diets, focusing on readily available and versatile ingredients, makes it an ideal choice for busy individuals seeking to make healthful changes without the need for drastic lifestyle overhauls.

The practicality of integrating the Mediterranean and DASH diets into daily life is underscored by their emphasis on foods that are not only nutritious but also widely accessible and easy to prepare. This approach supports sustainable dietary changes that can be maintained over the long term, a crucial aspect for those aiming to lower blood pressure, enhance heart health, and achieve weight loss without feeling restricted or overwhelmed by complicated meal plans. The simplicity of focusing on fresh produce, whole grains, and lean proteins, while limiting processed foods and high-sodium options, aligns with the busy lifestyles of many individuals, making it feasible to adopt healthier eating habits amidst a hectic schedule.

Moreover, the combined diet encourages culinary exploration and creativity, allowing for the incorporation of a broad spectrum of flavors and ingredients that cater to diverse palates and cultural preferences. This inclusivity not only enhances meal satisfaction but also facilitates adherence to the diet, as individuals are less likely to feel bored or constrained by their food choices. The Mediterranean-DASH diet fusion thus represents a versatile and adaptable eating plan that can accommodate various dietary needs and preferences, making it an appealing option for a wide audience.

The role of moderate physical activity, as recommended by both diets, cannot be overstated in its contribution to cardiovascular health and overall well-being. Regular exercise complements the dietary aspects of the Mediterranean and DASH diets by further reducing blood pressure, aiding in weight management, and improving metabolic health. This holistic approach to health underscores the importance of a balanced lifestyle that combines nutritious eating with physical activity, offering a comprehensive strategy for preventing hypertension, heart disease, and other chronic conditions.

Educational initiatives and resources that provide guidance on how to effectively combine the Mediterranean and DASH diets can play a significant role in helping individuals navigate the transition to healthier eating habits. Cooking classes, meal planning tools, and nutritional counseling are valuable supports that can demystify the process of adopting these dietary principles, making it more accessible to those with limited culinary experience or knowledge of nutrition. By offering practical tips and strategies for incorporating heart-healthy foods into daily meals, such resources can empower individuals to take proactive steps towards improving their health.

In conclusion, the fusion of the Mediterranean and DASH diets offers a powerful dietary approach for enhancing heart health, lowering blood pressure, and achieving sustainable weight loss. Its emphasis on whole foods, balanced nutrition, and the inclusion of moderate physical activity aligns with the goals of improving overall well-being and preventing chronic diseases. The practicality, flexibility, and inclusivity of this combined diet make it an attractive option for individuals seeking to make healthful changes to their eating habits, regardless of their culinary skills or nutritional knowledge. With the right support and resources, adopting the Mediterranean-DASH diet can be a rewarding journey towards a healthier, more vibrant life.

Understanding Hypertension and Heart Health

Hypertension, commonly known as high blood pressure, is a condition where the force of the blood against the artery walls is too high. Normally, blood pressure rises and falls throughout the day, but when it stays high over time, it can cause health problems. Hypertension is often labeled as a "silent killer" because it can be present for years without any symptoms, yet it can lead to serious health issues, including heart disease, stroke, and kidney failure.

Blood pressure is measured in millimeters of mercury (mm Hg) and is given by two numbers. The first, or top number, is the systolic pressure, which indicates the pressure in the arteries when the heart beats. The second, or bottom number, is the diastolic pressure, which shows the pressure in the arteries when the heart rests between beats. A normal blood pressure level is less than 120/80 mm Hg. Hypertension is defined as having a blood pressure higher than 130 over 80 mm Hg, measured on two different occasions.

The heart plays a crucial role in the body's circulatory system, pumping blood throughout the body to supply tissues with oxygen and nutrients. Hypertension can damage the heart in several ways. First, it can harden and narrow the arteries, limiting the flow of oxygen-rich blood to the heart muscle. This condition, known as coronary artery disease, can lead to chest pain, heart attack, or heart failure. Heart failure occurs when the heart cannot pump enough blood to meet the body's needs.

Moreover, hypertension forces the heart to work harder than normal. Over time, this extra effort can cause the heart muscle to thicken and become less efficient at pumping blood, a condition known as left ventricular hypertrophy. Eventually, this can lead to heart failure, where the heart is unable to pump effectively, leading to fluid buildup in the lungs and other parts of the body.

Preventing and managing hypertension is critical for maintaining heart health. Lifestyle changes such as eating a balanced diet low in sodium, maintaining a healthy weight, engaging in regular physical activity, limiting alcohol consumption, and avoiding tobacco use can help manage blood pressure. Additionally, the Mediterranean and DASH diets, which emphasize fruits, vegetables, whole grains, and lean proteins while limiting salt, saturated fats, and added sugars, have been shown to be effective in lowering blood pressure and improving heart health.

It's also important for individuals to regularly monitor their blood pressure and consult with healthcare providers to manage their condition effectively. In some cases, medication may be necessary to control hypertension and prevent complications. By understanding hypertension and taking steps to control it, individuals can significantly reduce their risk of heart disease and improve their overall health.

The Role of Diet in Lowering Blood Pressure

The Mediterranean and DASH diets play a pivotal role in lowering blood pressure, a key factor in preventing heart disease and stroke. Both diets emphasize the intake of fruits, vegetables, whole grains, and lean proteins, which are rich in nutrients that are essential for heart health. The DASH diet, specifically designed to combat hypertension, focuses on reducing sodium intake and increasing foods high in potassium, calcium, and magnesium—minerals that help lower blood pressure. The Mediterranean diet, rich in healthy fats like olive oil and omega-3 fatty acids from fish, contributes to improved arterial health and reduced inflammation, further supporting cardiovascular wellness.

Incorporating these dietary patterns into daily life can significantly reduce systolic and diastolic blood pressure. For instance, the DASH diet encourages the consumption of nuts, seeds, legumes, lean meats, and low-fat dairy, all while limiting salt, red meat, sweets, and beverages containing sugar. Similarly, the Mediterranean diet promotes a high intake of fruits, vegetables, whole grains, and olive oil, moderate consumption of fish and poultry, and minimal intake of dairy products, red meat, and sweets. Together, these diets offer a comprehensive approach to eating that not only lowers blood pressure but also supports overall heart health.

By focusing on whole foods and limiting processed and high-sodium foods, individuals can naturally decrease their blood pressure. This dietary approach, coupled with lifestyle modifications like regular physical activity, maintaining a healthy weight, and avoiding tobacco use, can lead to significant improvements in blood pressure control and overall cardiovascular health.

Manage Weight Loss

The Mediterranean and DASH diets, both celebrated for their cardiovascular benefits, also play a significant role in weight management. The essence of weight loss and maintenance lies in creating a sustainable calorie deficit while ensuring nutritional adequacy, a principle both diets adeptly incorporate through their focus on whole, nutrient-dense foods.

At the heart of the Mediterranean diet is an abundance of fruits, vegetables, whole grains, olive oil, and lean proteins, particularly fish. This diet emphasizes food quality and the pleasure of eating, encouraging meals to be savored and enjoyed, not just consumed for sustenance. The high fiber content of the diet, thanks to its focus on plant-based foods, contributes to satiety, helping to naturally reduce calorie intake without the need for calorie counting. The inclusion of healthy fats, primarily from olive oil and fish, not only supports heart health but also contributes to feeling full, further aiding in weight control.

Similarly, the DASH diet, designed primarily to combat hypertension, emphasizes fruits, vegetables, whole grains, and lean proteins, including fish, poultry, and beans. It is particularly noted for its low sodium recommendations, which not only support blood pressure management but also help prevent water retention, a common issue that can affect weight measurements. The DASH diet's emphasis on potassium-rich foods aids in balancing sodium levels in the body, further supporting healthy weight management. Like the Mediterranean diet, DASH promotes the intake of foods high in fiber and protein, both of which are essential for weight loss and maintenance due to their roles in satiety and metabolism.

Both diets advocate for minimal intake of processed foods, sweets, and red meats, which are often high in calories, saturated fats, and added sugars, contributing to weight gain and health issues when consumed in excess. By focusing on nutrient-dense, whole foods, these diets naturally align with the principles of weight management by promoting foods that are both filling and nutritious.

The synergy between the Mediterranean and DASH diets offers a comprehensive approach to eating that supports not only cardiovascular health but also weight management. By prioritizing whole foods, these diets naturally create a dietary pattern that is lower in calories but high in nutrients, making it easier for individuals to achieve and maintain a healthy weight without feeling deprived. This approach not only supports physical health but also enhances the enjoyment of food, a key factor in the long-term sustainability of any diet plan.

In summary, the Mediterranean and DASH diets contribute to weight management through their emphasis on whole, nutrient-dense foods that support satiety and nutritional adequacy. Their focus on quality, rather than just quantity, of food, aligns with the principles of healthy weight loss and maintenance, offering a sustainable and enjoyable path to achieving health goals.

Chapter 3: Allowed and Limited Foods

In the realm of the 5-Ingredient Mediterranean DASH Diet Cookbook, understanding the delineation between allowed foods and those to limit is pivotal for adhering to a diet that marries the heart-healthy benefits of the Mediterranean and DASH diets. This chapter systematically categorizes foods into those encouraged for daily consumption and those best consumed sparingly or avoided to maintain the diet's integrity, aimed at lowering blood pressure, improving heart health, and facilitating weight management.

Allowed Foods:
The cornerstone of this diet is a rich variety of whole, unprocessed foods known for their nutritional value and health benefits. Fruits and vegetables of all kinds are encouraged, providing a spectrum of vitamins, minerals, and fiber, essential for heart health and overall well-being. Whole grains, such as quinoa, farro, and whole wheat, are preferred for their fiber content, which aids in digestion and provides a steady energy source. Lean proteins, including fish, poultry, and plant-based options like beans and lentils, are emphasized for their ability to satisfy hunger and repair body tissues. Healthy fats, particularly those from olive oil, nuts, and seeds, are integral to this diet, offering cardiovascular benefits and aiding in the absorption of fat-soluble vitamins. Dairy products, when included, should be low-fat or fat-free to keep saturated fat intake in check.

Foods to Limit or Avoid:
In contrast, certain foods are to be limited or avoided to adhere to the diet's low-sodium, heart-healthy principles. High-sodium foods, such as processed meats, canned soups, and fast foods, are to be consumed sparingly, if at all, due to their link to hypertension. Sweets and sugary beverages, high in added sugars and empty calories, are discouraged, as they can contribute to weight gain and disrupt blood sugar levels. Full-fat dairy products and fatty cuts of meat are limited due to their high saturated fat content, which can negatively impact heart health. Lastly, alcohol intake should be moderate, aligning with the diet's emphasis on moderation and overall wellness.

Budget-Friendly Weekly Shopping List:
To implement this diet effectively, planning is key. A weekly shopping list that emphasizes the allowed foods while considering budget constraints can make adherence both feasible and enjoyable. This list includes a variety of fruits and vegetables, focusing on seasonal produce for cost-effectiveness; bulk purchases of whole grains; lean proteins, with a preference for plant-based options to reduce costs; and healthy fats, such as bulk nuts and olive oil purchased in larger containers. This approach ensures that the diet is both nutritionally adequate and financially sustainable.

Reading and Understanding Food Labels:
Equally important is the ability to read and understand food labels, which empowers individuals to make informed choices about the foods they include in their diet. Key points include identifying serving sizes, recognizing the amount of sodium, sugars, and saturated fat per

serving, and understanding the list of ingredients to avoid foods high in additives and preservatives. This knowledge is crucial for adhering to the Mediterranean DASH diet principles, ensuring that the choices made align with the goals of lowering blood pressure, improving heart health, and managing weight.

By focusing on allowed foods and understanding which foods to limit or avoid, individuals can navigate the Mediterranean DASH diet with confidence, enjoying a wide range of healthful, delicious foods that support their health goals. This chapter provides the foundation for making dietary choices that are in harmony with the principles of the Mediterranean and DASH diets, offering a path to improved well-being through mindful eating.

Allowed Foods

In adhering to the principles of the 5-Ingredient Mediterranean DASH Diet Cookbook, the focus is on whole, nutrient-dense foods that support heart health, weight management, and overall well-being. The allowed foods are categorized into groups that emphasize the consumption of fresh produce, lean proteins, whole grains, and healthy fats. Below is a detailed breakdown of these food categories:

Fruits: All fresh, frozen, or canned without added sugars. Examples include apples, bananas, berries, oranges, and pears.

Vegetables: Emphasizes a variety, including leafy greens, root vegetables, and legumes. Options like spinach, carrots, broccoli, and lentils are encouraged.

Whole Grains: Focus on grains that are minimally processed. Quinoa, brown rice, whole wheat pasta, and oats are excellent choices.

Lean Proteins: Incorporates both animal and plant sources. Fish, poultry, beans, and nuts are key for a balanced diet.

Healthy Fats: Sources of monounsaturated and polyunsaturated fats like olive oil, avocados, and seeds are essential.

Dairy: Opt for low-fat or fat-free options such as milk, yogurt, and cheese to reduce saturated fat intake.

This dietary approach limits processed foods, high-sodium items, and foods high in added sugars and saturated fats. By focusing on the allowed foods, individuals can enjoy a diverse and flavorful diet that supports their health goals without feeling restricted.

Foods to Limit or Avoid

In adhering to the principles of the 5-Ingredient Mediterranean DASH Diet Cookbook, it's crucial to recognize that while many foods support heart health, weight management, and overall well-being, there are certain foods and ingredients that should be limited or avoided. These foods, typically high in sodium, saturated fats, added sugars, and processed components, can counteract the benefits of the Mediterranean and DASH diets. Below is a detailed categorization of foods to limit or avoid to maintain the integrity of combining these two healthful diets:

Processed and High-Sodium Foods:
- Canned soups and vegetables with added salt
- Deli meats and sausages
- Salted snacks (chips, pretzels)
- Fast food items

Sweets and Sugary Beverages:
- Soda and sweetened drinks
- Candy and chocolate bars (except for dark chocolate in moderation)
- Pastries, cookies, and cakes
- Ice cream and other sugar-heavy desserts

High-Fat Dairy and Fatty Meats:
- Whole milk, cream, and full-fat cheese
- Butter and cream-based sauces
- Fatty cuts of beef, pork, and lamb
- Processed meats like bacon and hot dogs

Alcohol:
- Limit to moderate consumption as defined by dietary guidelines

Refined Grains:
- White bread and pasta
- Pastries made with refined flour
- White rice

Limiting or avoiding these foods can help in reducing the intake of unhealthy fats, added sugars, and excess sodium, which are known contributors to hypertension, weight gain, and cardiovascular diseases. By focusing on whole, nutrient-dense foods and minimizing the consumption of these restricted categories, individuals can enjoy the full spectrum of health benefits offered by the Mediterranean and DASH diet combination. This approach not only supports physical health but also promotes a sustainable and pleasurable eating pattern that can be maintained over time.

Budget-Friendly Weekly Shopping List

Fresh Produce

Avocados: 6 large
Bananas: 4 medium
Basil: 1 bunch (about 1 oz)
Beets: 2 medium (about 1 lb)
Blueberries: 1 pint (about 12 oz)
Broccoli: 2 heads (about 1 lb each)
Carrots: 4 medium (about 1 lb)
Cauliflower: 1 head (about 2 lbs)
Cucumbers: 4 medium
Eggplant: 1 medium (about 1 lb)
Garlic: 1 bulb
Grapes: 1 bunch (about 1 lb)
Kale: 1 bunch (about 8 oz)
Lemons: 4 medium
Lettuce (Arugula, Spinach, etc.): 2 bags (about 5 oz each)
Mushrooms: 2 cups sliced (about 8 oz)
Peaches: 2 medium
Radishes: 1 bunch (about 8 oz)
Red Bell Peppers: 2 large
Tomatoes: 8 medium (about 1.5 lbs)
Zucchini: 4 medium (about 1 lb)

Dairy

Almond Milk or Regular Milk: 1 quart
Cottage Cheese: 16 oz container
Feta Cheese: 8 oz block
Goat Cheese: 8 oz block
Greek Yogurt: 32 oz container (plain or flavored)
Ricotta Cheese: 15 oz container
Eggs: 1 dozen large
Parmesan Cheese: 8 oz block

Grains

Bagels: 1 package (6 bagels)

Chickpeas (Canned or Dry): 2 cans (15 oz each) or 1 lb dry
Farro or Quinoa: 1 lb bag
Oats: 18 oz bag
Pasta: 1 lb package (your choice)
Whole Wheat Tortillas or Wraps: 1 package (8 wraps)

Protein

Chicken Breast: 1.5 lbs (boneless, skinless)
Lentils: 1 lb bag (dry)
Salmon Fillets: 1 lb (about 2 fillets)
Shrimp: 1 lb (fresh or frozen, peeled and deveined)
Tuna (Canned): 2 cans (5 oz each)

Canned/Packaged Goods

Almond Butter: 16 oz jar
Balsamic Vinegar: 16 oz bottle
Hummus: 10 oz container
Olive Oil: 16 oz bottle
Peanut Butter: 16 oz jar
Pesto: 6 oz jar
Tomato Sauce: 15 oz jar

Nuts/Seeds

Almonds: 8 oz bag (whole or sliced)
Chia Seeds: 12 oz bag
Walnuts: 8 oz bag (halves or pieces)

Spices/Condiments

Cinnamon: 2 oz jar
Dried Herbs (Oregano, Thyme, etc.): 1 oz jar each
Salt: 26 oz container
Black Pepper: 4 oz container
Honey: 12 oz jar

Weekly Meal Plan Suggestions

Breakfasts: Rotate between Avocado and Egg Toast, Berry Yogurt Parfait, Chia Seed Pudding, and other recipes.
Lunches: Enjoy salads, wraps, and chickpea dishes.
Dinners: Try different protein options with veggies and pasta.
Snacks: Include Greek Salad Skewers, Roasted Chickpeas, and other appetizers.
Desserts: Treat yourself with Almond Butter Cookies and other sweet options.

Tips

Ingredient Variations: Feel free to substitute ingredients based on personal preferences or seasonal availability (e.g., swap fruits or greens).
Bulk Buying: Purchase grains, nuts, and seeds in bulk for cost savings.

Reading and Understanding Food Labels

Reading and understanding food labels is an essential skill for anyone looking to maintain a healthy diet, especially when following the principles of the Mediterranean DASH Diet. Food labels provide a wealth of information about the nutritional content of food items, helping individuals make informed choices that align with their health goals. This is particularly important for managing sodium intake, understanding the balance of macronutrients, and avoiding foods high in added sugars and unhealthy fats which are pivotal aspects of both the Mediterranean and DASH diets.

The first component of a food label to pay attention to is the serving size. This information is critical because all the nutritional values listed on the label refer to this specific amount of food. Misinterpreting serving sizes can lead to underestimating the intake of calories, sodium, and fats, which can hinder the management of blood pressure and weight loss efforts. It's also beneficial to compare the serving size to the portion you actually consume and adjust the nutritional information accordingly.

Next, the calories section of the label indicates the amount of energy provided by one serving of the food. Managing caloric intake is crucial for weight maintenance and loss, a common objective for followers of the Mediterranean DASH Diet. Lowering calorie intake, while ensuring nutritional adequacy, supports weight loss and reduces the risk of chronic diseases associated with obesity.

Sodium content is another critical section of the food label, especially for individuals concerned with lowering blood pressure. The Mediterranean DASH Diet emphasizes low sodium intake to manage hypertension. Food labels help identify high-sodium foods to limit or avoid and find lower-sodium alternatives that are better suited for heart health.

Furthermore, the label lists macronutrients, including total fat, saturated fat, trans fat, cholesterol, carbohydrates, dietary fiber, total sugars, and added sugars. For adherents of the

Mediterranean DASH Diet, focusing on foods with healthy fats, such as monounsaturated and polyunsaturated fats, and high in fiber is essential. These nutrients contribute to heart health, aid in digestion, and can help with feeling full longer, which assists in weight management. Limiting saturated fats, added sugars, and cholesterol is also crucial for cardiovascular health.

Lastly, vitamins and minerals section on the label, such as potassium, calcium, and magnesium, are of particular interest. The DASH diet, in part, focuses on increasing the intake of these nutrients to counteract the effects of sodium and support overall heart health. Identifying foods high in these beneficial nutrients can help individuals meet their daily recommended intakes.

In essence, reading and understanding food labels empowers individuals to make choices that align with the dietary principles of the Mediterranean DASH Diet. It enables the identification of nutrient-dense foods that support heart health, weight management, and overall well-being. By paying close attention to serving sizes, calories, sodium, macronutrients, and vitamins and minerals, individuals can navigate their dietary choices more effectively, ensuring they align with their health objectives.

Chapter 4: Recipes

Breakfast Recipes

Avocado and Egg Toast

Preparation Time: 10 minutes
Cooking Time: 5 minutes
Ingredients:
- 1 ripe avocado
- 2 slices of whole-grain bread
- 2 eggs
- Salt and pepper to taste
- Red pepper flakes (optional)

Instructions:
1. Toast the whole-grain bread slices to your preferred level of crispiness.
2. While the bread is toasting, mash the ripe avocado in a small bowl and season with salt and pepper. Set aside.
3. In a non-stick skillet, cook the eggs to your liking; sunny side up or scrambled works well for this recipe.
4. Spread the mashed avocado evenly on each slice of toasted bread, top each with an egg, and sprinkle with red pepper flakes if desired.

Macronutrients:
- **Kcal:** 320
- **Carbs:** 29g
- **Protein:** 12g
- **Fat:** 18g
- **Potassium:** 487mg
- **Calcium:** 52mg
- **Magnesium:** 58mg

Ingredient Variation Tip: For an extra protein boost, add a slice of smoked salmon under the egg. This not only increases the protein content but also adds omega-3 fatty acids, beneficial for heart health.

Banana Oat Pancakes

Preparation Time: 10 minutes
Cooking Time: 15 minutes
Ingredients:
- 2 ripe bananas
- 1 cup rolled oats
- 2 large eggs
- 1/2 teaspoon baking powder
- 1/4 cup milk (any kind)

Instructions:
1. In a blender, combine the bananas, rolled oats, eggs, baking powder, and milk. Blend until the mixture is smooth and the oats are fully broken down.
2. Heat a non-stick skillet over medium heat. Pour 1/4 cup of the batter onto the skillet for each pancake. Cook until bubbles form on the surface, then flip and cook until golden brown on the other side, about 2-3 minutes per side.
3. Repeat with the remaining batter, adding more milk if the batter becomes too thick.
4. Serve the pancakes warm.

Macronutrients:
- **Kcal:** 320
- **Carbs:** 58g
- **Protein:** 11g
- **Fat:** 7g
- **Potassium:** 422mg
- **Calcium:** 60mg
- **Magnesium:** 81mg

Ingredient Variation Tip: For a gluten-free version, ensure the rolled oats are certified gluten-free. To add a protein boost, blend in a scoop of your favorite protein powder.

Berry Yogurt Parfait

Preparation Time: 10 minutes

Cooking Time: 0 minutes

Ingredients:
- 1 cup Greek yogurt, low-fat
- ½ cup mixed berries (strawberries, blueberries, raspberries)
- ¼ cup granola, low-sodium
- 1 tablespoon honey
- A pinch of cinnamon (optional)

Instructions:
1. In a serving glass or bowl, layer half of the Greek yogurt at the bottom.
2. Add a layer of mixed berries over the yogurt.
3. Sprinkle half of the granola over the berries and drizzle with half of the honey. If using, sprinkle a tiny bit of cinnamon.
4. Repeat the layers with the remaining ingredients, starting with yogurt and ending with a drizzle of honey and a sprinkle of cinnamon.

Macronutrients:
- **Kcal:** 290
- **Carbs:** 42g
- **Protein:** 20g
- **Fat:** 6g
- **Potassium:** 345mg
- **Calcium:** 190mg
- **Magnesium:** 30mg

Ingredient Variation Tip: For a vegan version, substitute Greek yogurt with a plant-based yogurt alternative. Maple syrup can be used in place of honey for a different sweetness profile.

Caprese Avocado Toast

Preparation Time: 10 minutes

Cooking Time: 0 minutes

Ingredients:
- 2 slices of whole-grain bread
- 1 ripe avocado
- 4 slices of fresh mozzarella cheese
- 2 ripe tomatoes, sliced
- Fresh basil leaves
- Salt and pepper to taste

Instructions:
1. Toast the whole-grain bread slices to your preferred level of crispiness.
2. While the bread is toasting, peel and pit the avocado. In a small bowl, mash the avocado with a fork until it reaches a smooth consistency. Season with salt and pepper to taste.
3. Spread the mashed avocado evenly over the toasted bread slices. Place two slices of fresh mozzarella cheese on each piece of toast.
4. Top the mozzarella with sliced tomatoes and fresh basil leaves. Add an additional sprinkle of salt and pepper if desired.

Macronutrients:
- **Kcal:** 350
- **Carbs:** 27g
- **Protein:** 12g
- **Fat:** 22g
- **Potassium:** 487mg
- **Calcium:** 200mg
- **Magnesium:** 45mg

Ingredient Variation Tip: For an extra burst of flavor, drizzle a small amount of balsamic glaze over the top of your Caprese Avocado Toast before serving.

Chia Seed Pudding

Preparation time: 5 minutes

Cooking time: 0 minutes (requires at least 4 hours of refrigeration)

Ingredients:
- 1/4 cup chia seeds
- 1 cup unsweetened almond milk
- 1 tablespoon maple syrup (or honey)
- 1/2 teaspoon vanilla extract
- Fresh berries for topping

Instructions:
1. In a medium bowl, whisk together the chia seeds, almond milk, maple syrup, and vanilla extract until well combined.
2. Pour the mixture into a jar or a glass container and refrigerate for at least 4 hours, preferably overnight, until it has thickened and reached a pudding-like consistency.
3. Once set, stir the pudding. If it's too thick, you can add a little more almond milk to reach your desired consistency.
4. Serve the chia seed pudding topped with fresh berries of your choice.

Macronutrients:
- **kcal:** 210
- **Carbs:** 24g
- **Protein:** 5g
- **Fat:** 11g
- **Potassium:** 103mg
- **Calcium:** 351mg
- **Magnesium:** 95mg

Ingredient Variation Tip: For a tropical twist, replace almond milk with coconut milk and top with fresh mango or pineapple.

Cinnamon Apple Oatmeal

Preparation Time: 5 minutes

Cooking Time: 10 minutes

Ingredients:
- 1 cup rolled oats
- 2 cups water or milk (for a creamier texture)
- 1 large apple, peeled and diced
- 1 teaspoon ground cinnamon
- 1 tablespoon honey or maple syrup (optional for sweetness)

Instructions:
1. In a medium saucepan, bring the 2 cups of water or milk to a boil. Add the rolled oats and reduce the heat to a simmer. Cook, stirring occasionally, for about 5 minutes.
2. While the oats are cooking, add the diced apple and ground cinnamon to the saucepan. Stir well to combine.
3. Continue to cook the mixture for another 5 minutes, or until the oats are soft and have absorbed most of the liquid.
4. Remove from heat and let it sit for 2 minutes to thicken. Serve warm, drizzled with honey or maple syrup if desired.

Macronutrients:
- **Kcal:** 350
- **Carbs:** 60g
- **Protein:** 10g
- **Fat:** 5g
- **Potassium:** 240mg
- **Calcium:** 20mg
- **Magnesium:** 80mg

Ingredient Variation Tip: For an added nutritional boost and texture, sprinkle a tablespoon of chia seeds or flaxseeds into the oatmeal while cooking.

Cottage Cheese and Fruit Bowl

Preparation Time: 5 minutes

Cooking Time: 0 minutes

Ingredients:
- 1 cup low-fat cottage cheese
- 1/2 cup mixed fresh berries (such as strawberries, blueberries, and raspberries)
- 1/4 cup sliced almonds
- 1 tablespoon honey
- A pinch of cinnamon (optional)

Instructions:
1. Place the cottage cheese at the bottom of a serving bowl.
2. Top the cottage cheese with the mixed fresh berries.
3. Sprinkle the sliced almonds over the berries and cottage cheese.
4. Drizzle honey over the top and add a pinch of cinnamon if desired. Serve immediately.

Macronutrients:
- **Kcal:** 350
- **Carbs:** 34g
- **Protein:** 28g
- **Fat:** 10g
- **Potassium:** 200mg
- **Calcium:** 150mg
- **Magnesium:** 50mg

Ingredient Variation Tip: For a tropical twist, substitute the berries with a mix of diced mango, pineapple, and kiwi.

Egg and Spinach Wrap

Preparation Time: 10 minutes

Cooking Time: 5 minutes

Ingredients:
- 1 large egg
- 1 cup fresh spinach
- 1 whole wheat tortilla wrap
- 1 tablespoon feta cheese, crumbled
- 1 teaspoon olive oil

Instructions:
1. Heat the olive oil in a non-stick skillet over medium heat. Add the spinach and sauté until just wilted, about 1-2 minutes. Remove from skillet and set aside.
2. In the same skillet, crack the egg and cook to your liking, either scrambled or sunny-side up.
3. Warm the whole wheat tortilla wrap in the microwave for about 10 seconds to make it pliable.
4. Place the cooked egg, sautéed spinach, and crumbled feta cheese on the tortilla. Fold the bottom up, then fold the sides in, rolling it securely.

Macronutrients:
- **Kcal:** 250
- **Carbs:** 18g
- **Protein:** 12g
- **Fat:** 15g
- **Potassium:** 200mg
- **Calcium:** 150mg
- **Magnesium:** 50mg

Ingredient Variation Tip: For a vegan version, substitute the egg with a scrambled tofu mix and use a dairy-free cheese alternative.

Feta and Tomato Omelette

Preparation Time: 10 minutes

Cooking Time: 10 minutes

Ingredients:
- 2 large eggs
- 1/4 cup crumbled feta cheese
- 1/2 tomato, diced
- 1 tablespoon olive oil
- Salt and pepper to taste

Instructions:
1. In a medium bowl, whisk the eggs until fully blended. Season with a pinch of salt and pepper.
2. Heat the olive oil in a non-stick skillet over medium heat. Add the diced tomato and sauté for 2 minutes until slightly softened.
3. Pour the whisked eggs over the tomatoes, tilting the pan to ensure an even spread. Cook for about 3 minutes, or until the eggs start to set around the edges.
4. Sprinkle the feta cheese over half of the omelette. Using a spatula, gently fold the other half over the cheese. Cook for another 2 minutes, or until the cheese is slightly melted and the eggs are cooked to your liking.

Macronutrients:
- **Kcal:** 290
- **Carbs:** 4g
- **Protein:** 16g
- **Fat:** 24g
- **Potassium:** 210mg
- **Calcium:** 150mg
- **Magnesium:** 30mg

Ingredient Variation Tip: For a touch of Mediterranean flavor, add a few leaves of fresh basil or spinach to the omelette before folding.

Greek Yogurt with Honey and Nuts

Preparation Time: 5 minutes

Cooking Time: 0 minutes

Ingredients:
- 1 cup Greek yogurt (plain, non-fat)
- 2 tablespoons honey
- 1/4 cup mixed nuts (almonds, walnuts, and pistachios), roughly chopped
- 1/2 teaspoon ground cinnamon (optional)
- Fresh berries for topping (optional)

Instructions:
1. In a serving bowl, place the Greek yogurt.
2. Drizzle the honey over the yogurt evenly.
3. Sprinkle the chopped nuts on top of the honey. If desired, add a dash of ground cinnamon for extra flavor.
4. Garnish with fresh berries if using. Serve immediately for a refreshing and nutritious breakfast.

Macronutrients:
- **Kcal:** 310
- **Carbs:** 35g
- **Protein:** 20g
- **Fat:** 10g
- **Potassium:** 240mg
- **Calcium:** 150mg
- **Magnesium:** 45mg

Ingredient Variation Tip: For a vegan version, substitute Greek yogurt with a plant-based yogurt alternative and use maple syrup instead of honey.

Mediterranean Breakfast Burrito

Preparation Time: 10 minutes
Cooking Time: 10 minutes
Ingredients:
- 2 whole wheat tortillas
- 4 eggs, beaten
- 1 ripe avocado, sliced
- 1/2 cup cooked black beans, rinsed and drained
- 1/4 cup crumbled feta cheese
- Salt and pepper to taste

Instructions:

1. Heat a non-stick skillet over medium heat. Add the beaten eggs and scramble until fully cooked, about 3-4 minutes. Season with salt and pepper to taste. Remove from heat and set aside.
2. Warm the whole wheat tortillas in the microwave for about 20 seconds or until soft and pliable.
3. Divide the scrambled eggs evenly among the tortillas. Top each with sliced avocado, black beans, and crumbled feta cheese.
4. Roll up the tortillas tightly to form burritos. If desired, you can lightly grill the burritos on a skillet over medium heat for 1-2 minutes on each side to crisp the tortillas.

Macronutrients:
- **Calories:** 350 kcal
- **Carbs:** 35 g
- **Protein:** 18 g
- **Fat:** 18 g
- **Potassium:** 600 mg
- **Calcium:** 150 mg
- **Magnesium:** 45 mg

Ingredient Variation Tip: For a twist, add a spoonful of salsa inside the burrito or swap the black beans for chickpeas for a different flavor profile.

Mushroom and Feta Scramble

Preparation Time: 10 minutes

Cooking Time: 10 minutes

Ingredients:
- 4 large eggs
- 1 cup sliced mushrooms
- 1/4 cup crumbled feta cheese
- 2 tablespoons olive oil
- Salt and pepper to taste

Instructions:

1. Heat the olive oil in a non-stick skillet over medium heat. Add the sliced mushrooms and sauté until they are soft and browned, about 5-7 minutes. Season with a pinch of salt and pepper.
2. In a bowl, whisk the eggs with a pinch of salt and pepper until well combined. Pour the eggs over the sautéed mushrooms in the skillet.
3. Allow the eggs to set for a minute before gently stirring to create a scramble. Cook to your desired level of doneness.
4. Sprinkle the crumbled feta cheese over the eggs and mushrooms. Stir gently to mix. Serve immediately.

Macronutrients:
- **Kcal:** 300
- **Carbs:** 2g
- **Protein:** 18g
- **Fat:** 24g
- **Potassium:** 200mg
- **Calcium:** 150mg
- **Magnesium:** 30mg

Ingredient Variation Tip: For a touch of green, add a handful of spinach to the skillet when sautéing the mushrooms. It will add color, nutrients, and a slight earthy flavor that complements the feta cheese beautifully.

Olive and Herb Frittata

Preparation Time: 10 minutes
Cooking Time: 15 minutes
Ingredients:
- 6 large eggs
- 1/4 cup milk (low-fat for a healthier option)
- 1/2 cup chopped fresh herbs (such as parsley, basil, and chives)
- 1/2 cup diced olives (preferably Kalamata)
- 1 tablespoon olive oil
- Salt and pepper to taste

Instructions:
1. Preheat your oven to 375°F (190°C). In a medium bowl, whisk together the eggs, milk, salt, and pepper until well combined. Stir in the chopped herbs and diced olives.
2. Heat the olive oil in an oven-safe skillet over medium heat. Once hot, pour the egg mixture into the skillet, stirring gently to ensure the olives and herbs are evenly distributed.
3. Cook without stirring for about 2-3 minutes until the edges start to set. Then, transfer the skillet to the preheated oven.
4. Bake for 10-12 minutes, or until the frittata is set and lightly golden on top. Remove from the oven, let it cool for a couple of minutes, then slice and serve.

Macronutrients:
- **Kcal:** 220
- **Carbs:** 2g
- **Protein:** 14g
- **Fat:** 17g
- **Potassium:** 210mg
- **Calcium:** 60mg
- **Magnesium:** 20mg

Ingredient Variation Tip: For a dairy-free version, substitute the milk with unsweetened almond milk.

Quinoa Breakfast Bowl

Preparation Time: 5 minutes

Cooking Time: 15 minutes

Ingredients:
- 1 cup quinoa
- 2 cups water
- 1/2 cup sliced strawberries
- 1/4 cup chopped almonds
- 2 tablespoons honey

Instructions:
1. Rinse 1 cup of quinoa under cold water until the water runs clear. Combine the rinsed quinoa and 2 cups of water in a medium saucepan. Bring to a boil over high heat, then reduce the heat to low, cover, and simmer for about 15 minutes, or until the quinoa is cooked and water is absorbed.
2. Remove the quinoa from the heat and let it sit, covered, for 5 minutes. Fluff it with a fork to separate the grains.
3. Divide the cooked quinoa into bowls. Top each bowl with an equal amount of sliced strawberries and chopped almonds.
4. Drizzle each bowl with honey before serving.

Macronutrients:
- **Kcal:** 235
- **Carbs:** 39g
- **Protein:** 6g
- **Fat:** 5g
- **Potassium:** 320mg
- **Calcium:** 50mg
- **Magnesium:** 89mg

Ingredient Variation Tip: For a tropical twist, replace strawberries with diced mango or pineapple and almonds with macadamia nuts.

Smoked Salmon Bagel

Preparation Time: 10 minutes

Cooking Time: 0 minutes

Ingredients:
- 1 whole grain bagel, halved
- 2 oz smoked salmon
- 2 tbsp cream cheese, low-fat
- 1 tbsp capers
- 2 slices of red onion

Instructions:
1. Toast the bagel halves until they are lightly browned and crispy.
2. Spread 1 tablespoon of low-fat cream cheese on each half of the toasted bagel.
3. Place 1 ounce of smoked salmon on top of the cream cheese on each bagel half.
4. Garnish each half with capers and slices of red onion. Serve immediately.

Macronutrients:
- **Kcal:** 360
- **Carbs:** 44g
- **Protein:** 22g
- **Fat:** 12g
- **Potassium:** 330mg
- **Calcium:** 60mg
- **Magnesium:** 48mg

Ingredient Variation Tip: For a dairy-free option, substitute cream cheese with avocado spread. This not only adds a creamy texture but also provides healthy fats.

Spinach and Feta Muffins

Preparation Time: 10 minutes

Cooking Time: 15 minutes

Ingredients:
- 1 cup whole wheat flour
- 2 teaspoons baking powder
- 2 eggs
- 1 cup spinach, chopped
- 1/2 cup feta cheese, crumbled

Instructions:
1. Preheat your oven to 350°F (175°C) and line a muffin tin with paper liners or lightly grease it.
2. In a large bowl, mix together the whole wheat flour and baking powder. In a separate bowl, beat the eggs and then add the chopped spinach and crumbled feta cheese, mixing until just combined.
3. Add the wet ingredients to the dry ingredients, stirring until the mixture is just combined. Be careful not to overmix.
4. Divide the batter evenly among the muffin cups, filling each about two-thirds full. Bake in the preheated oven for 15 minutes, or until a toothpick inserted into the center of a muffin comes out clean.

Macronutrients:
- **Kcal:** 150
- **Carbs:** 18g
- **Protein:** 8g
- **Fat:** 6g
- **Potassium:** 125mg
- **Calcium:** 100mg
- **Magnesium:** 30mg

Ingredient Variation Tip: For a gluten-free version, substitute the whole wheat flour with almond flour or another gluten-free flour blend. Additionally, adding a few diced sun-dried tomatoes to the batter.

Tomato Basil Bruschetta

Preparation Time: 10 minutes

Cooking Time: 0 minutes

Ingredients:
- 4 large ripe tomatoes, diced
- 1/4 cup fresh basil leaves, chopped
- 2 tablespoons extra virgin olive oil
- 1 clove garlic, minced
- 1 loaf whole-grain baguette, sliced and toasted

Instructions:
1. In a medium mixing bowl, combine the diced tomatoes, chopped basil, extra virgin olive oil, and minced garlic. Stir the mixture gently until all the ingredients are well combined.
2. Allow the tomato mixture to sit for about 5 minutes to marinate, letting the flavors meld together.
3. Spoon the tomato mixture generously onto the slices of toasted baguette.
4. Serve immediately for the best flavor and texture.

Macronutrients:
- **kcal:** 150 per serving
- **Carbs:** 18g
- **Protein:** 4g
- **Fat:** 7g
- **Potassium:** 237mg
- **Calcium:** 35mg
- **Magnesium:** 22mg

Ingredient Variation Tip: For a protein boost, add a sprinkle of crumbled feta cheese or diced mozzarella on top of the bruschetta before serving. This not only adds a creamy texture but also complements the fresh flavors of the tomato and basil beautifully.

Veggie and Hummus Wrap

Preparation Time: 10 minutes

Cooking Time: 0 minutes

Ingredients:
- 2 whole grain tortillas
- 1/2 cup hummus
- 1 cup mixed greens (spinach, arugula, or lettuce)
- 1/2 cucumber, thinly sliced
- 1/2 bell pepper, thinly sliced

Instructions:
1. Lay out the whole grain tortillas on a flat surface. Spread a quarter cup of hummus evenly over each tortilla, leaving a small border around the edge.
2. Distribute the mixed greens across the center of each tortilla on top of the hummus.
3. Arrange the cucumber and bell pepper slices evenly over the greens.
4. Carefully roll up the tortillas tightly, starting from one edge and working your way to the other. Slice each wrap in half diagonally and serve immediately.

Macronutrients:
- **Kcal:** 250
- **Carbs:** 35g
- **Protein:** 8g
- **Fat:** 9g
- **Potassium:** 297mg
- **Calcium:** 75mg
- **Magnesium:** 30mg

Ingredient Variation Tip: For a gluten-free option, substitute whole grain tortillas with gluten-free tortillas. To add more protein, include slices of grilled chicken or turkey breast.

Yogurt and Granola Bowl

Preparation Time: 5 minutes

Cooking Time: 0 minutes

Ingredients:
- 1 cup low-fat Greek yogurt
- 1/2 cup granola (look for a low-sodium variety)
- 1/2 cup mixed berries (such as strawberries, blueberries, and raspberries)
- 1 tablespoon honey (optional)
- A pinch of cinnamon (optional)

Instructions:
1. In a bowl, layer the Greek yogurt at the bottom.
2. Sprinkle the granola evenly over the yogurt.
3. Add the mixed berries on top of the granola.
4. Drizzle with honey and a pinch of cinnamon for added flavor, if desired.

Macronutrients:
- **Kcal:** 350
- **Carbs:** 45g
- **Protein:** 20g
- **Fat:** 8g
- **Potassium:** 250mg
- **Calcium:** 150mg
- **Magnesium:** 30mg

Ingredient Variation Tip: For a vegan option, substitute Greek yogurt with a plant-based yogurt. You can also experiment with different types of fruit based on seasonal availability or personal preference.

Zucchini and Egg Muffins

Preparation Time: 10 minutes

Cooking Time: 15 minutes

Ingredients:
- 1 medium zucchini, grated
- 6 large eggs
- 1/2 cup feta cheese, crumbled
- 1/4 cup fresh basil, chopped
- Salt and pepper to taste

Instructions:
1. Preheat your oven to 375°F (190°C) and lightly grease a muffin tin.
2. In a large bowl, beat the eggs. Add the grated zucchini, feta cheese, chopped basil, and season with salt and pepper. Mix well to combine.
3. Pour the mixture into the prepared muffin tin, filling each cup about 3/4 full.
4. Bake in the preheated oven for 15 minutes, or until the muffins are set and lightly golden on top. Allow to cool for a few minutes before removing from the tin.

Macronutrients:
- **Kcal:** 150
- **Carbs:** 2g
- **Protein:** 9g
- **Fat:** 11g
- **Potassium:** 125mg
- **Calcium:** 90mg
- **Magnesium:** 15mg

Ingredient Variation Tip: For a different flavor profile, try substituting the feta cheese with goat cheese and the basil with spinach. This not only introduces a new taste but also adds a different set of nutrients.

Lunch Recipes

Artichoke and White Bean Salad

Preparation Time: 10 minutes
Cooking Time: 0 minutes
Ingredients:
- 1 can (14 ounces) artichoke hearts, drained and chopped
- 1 can (15 ounces) white beans (such as cannellini or great northern), rinsed and drained
- 2 tablespoons extra virgin olive oil
- 2 tablespoons lemon juice
- Salt and pepper to taste
Instructions:
1. In a large bowl, combine the chopped artichoke hearts and rinsed white beans.
2. Drizzle the extra virgin olive oil and lemon juice over the artichoke and bean mixture. Gently toss to ensure all ingredients are well coated.
3. Season the salad with salt and pepper to taste. Mix again to distribute the seasoning evenly.
4. Let the salad sit for about 5 minutes to allow the flavors to meld together before serving. Can be served chilled or at room temperature.
Macronutrients:
- **Kcal:** 200
- **Carbs:** 30g
- **Protein:** 8g
- **Fat:** 7g
- **Potassium:** 400mg
- **Calcium:** 80mg
- **Magnesium:** 75mg
Ingredient Variation Tip: For an added crunch and a nutty flavor, sprinkle some toasted pine nuts or slivered almonds over the salad before serving.

Balsamic Chicken and Veggie Skewers

Preparation Time: 10 minutes
Cooking Time: 10 minutes
Ingredients:
- 1 lb chicken breast, cut into 1-inch pieces
- 2 bell peppers, any color, cut into 1-inch pieces
- 1 zucchini, cut into 1-inch slices
- 1/4 cup balsamic vinegar
- 2 tablespoons olive oil
- Salt and pepper to taste
Instructions:
1. Preheat your grill to medium-high heat. In a large bowl, whisk together the balsamic vinegar, olive oil, salt, and pepper. Add the chicken pieces to the bowl and toss to coat evenly.
2. Thread the chicken, bell peppers, and zucchini onto skewers, alternating between the chicken and vegetables.
3. Place the skewers on the grill and cook for about 5 minutes on each side, or until the chicken is fully cooked and the vegetables are tender.
4. Remove from grill and let rest for a couple of minutes before serving.
Macronutrients:
- **Kcal:** 220
- **Carbs:** 8g
- **Protein:** 26g
- **Fat:** 9g
- **Potassium:** 500mg
- **Calcium:** 20mg
- **Magnesium:** 30mg
Ingredient Variation Tip: For a vegetarian option, substitute chicken with firm tofu or halloumi cheese. Ensure to press the tofu to remove excess water before marinating.

Chickpea and Spinach Stew

Preparation Time: 5 minutes

Cooking Time: 15 minutes

Ingredients:
- 1 can (15 oz) chickpeas, rinsed and drained
- 2 cups fresh spinach
- 1 large onion, diced
- 2 cloves garlic, minced
- 1 tsp olive oil

Instructions:
1. Heat the olive oil in a large pot over medium heat. Add the diced onion and minced garlic, sautéing until the onion becomes translucent, about 3-4 minutes.
2. Add the chickpeas to the pot and cook for another 5 minutes, stirring occasionally.
3. Stir in the fresh spinach and continue to cook until the spinach has wilted, about 2-3 minutes.
4. Add 2 cups of water to the pot, bring to a boil, then reduce the heat and simmer for 5 minutes. Season with salt and pepper to taste.

Macronutrients:
- **Kcal:** 210
- **Carbs:** 35g
- **Protein:** 11g
- **Fat:** 4g
- **Potassium:** 474mg
- **Calcium:** 80mg
- **Magnesium:** 79mg

Ingredient Variation Tip: For a richer flavor, add a teaspoon of smoked paprika or cumin when sautéing the onions and garlic.

Cucumber and Feta Salad

Preparation Time: 5 minutes

Cooking Time: 0 minutes

Ingredients:
- 2 large cucumbers, thinly sliced
- 1/2 cup feta cheese, crumbled
- 2 tablespoons olive oil
- 1 tablespoon lemon juice
- Salt and pepper to taste

Instructions:
1. In a large mixing bowl, combine the thinly sliced cucumbers and crumbled feta cheese.
2. In a small bowl, whisk together the olive oil and lemon juice until well combined. Season with salt and pepper to taste.
3. Pour the olive oil and lemon juice dressing over the cucumber and feta mixture. Toss gently to ensure all the slices are evenly coated.
4. Serve immediately, or chill in the refrigerator for about 15 minutes before serving for a refreshing touch.

Macronutrients:
- **Kcal:** 180
- **Carbs:** 6g
- **Protein:** 5g
- **Fat:** 15g
- **Potassium:** 230mg
- **Calcium:** 130mg
- **Magnesium:** 22mg

Ingredient Variation Tip: For an added crunch and nutritional boost, sprinkle some chopped walnuts or almonds over the salad before serving.

Eggplant and Tomato Stack

Preparation Time: 10 minutes
Cooking Time: 10 minutes
Ingredients:
- 1 large eggplant, sliced into 1/2-inch rounds
- 2 large tomatoes, sliced
- 1/4 cup low-fat ricotta cheese
- 2 tablespoons fresh basil, chopped
- Salt and pepper to taste

Instructions:
1. Preheat a grill or grill pan over medium heat. Season the eggplant slices with salt and pepper, and grill for about 4-5 minutes on each side, or until tender and grill marks appear.
2. On a serving plate, layer a slice of grilled eggplant, then a slice of tomato, and a teaspoon of ricotta cheese. Repeat the layering process until all ingredients are used, finishing with a dollop of ricotta on top.
3. Garnish the stack with fresh basil. Serve immediately or at room temperature.
4. For a richer flavor, you can drizzle a little balsamic glaze over the top before serving.

Macronutrients:
- **Kcal:** 180
- **Carbs:** 22g
- **Protein:** 9g
- **Fat:** 8g
- **Potassium:** 676mg
- **Calcium:** 150mg
- **Magnesium:** 55mg

Ingredient Variation Tip: For a vegan version, substitute ricotta cheese with a vegan almond or cashew cheese. To add a crunchy texture, sprinkle some toasted pine nuts or walnuts on top before serving.

Farro and Veggie Bowl

Preparation Time: 10 minutes
Cooking Time: 15 minutes
Ingredients:
- 1 cup farro
- 2 cups vegetable broth
- 1 cup cherry tomatoes, halved
- 1 cup cucumber, diced
- 1/4 cup red onion, finely chopped

Instructions:
1. Rinse the farro under cold water until the water runs clear. In a medium saucepan, combine the farro and vegetable broth. Bring to a boil over high heat, then reduce the heat to low, cover, and simmer for about 15 minutes, or until the farro is tender and the broth is absorbed.
2. While the farro is cooking, prepare the vegetables. Halve the cherry tomatoes, dice the cucumber, and finely chop the red onion.
3. Once the farro is cooked, fluff it with a fork and let it cool for a few minutes. Then, in a large mixing bowl, combine the cooked farro with the cherry tomatoes, cucumber, and red onion. Toss everything together until well mixed.
4. Serve the farro and veggie bowl either warm or at room temperature. If desired, you can add a drizzle of olive oil and a squeeze of lemon juice for extra flavor.

Macronutrients:
- **Kcal:** 320
- **Carbs:** 66g
- **Protein:** 9g
- **Fat:** 2g
- **Potassium:** 410mg
- **Calcium:** 30mg
- **Magnesium:** 60mg

Garbanzo Bean Salad

Preparation Time: 10 minutes
Cooking Time: 0 minutes
Ingredients:
- 1 can (15 oz) garbanzo beans (chickpeas), drained and rinsed
- 1 large cucumber, diced
- 1/2 red onion, finely chopped
- 1/4 cup fresh parsley, chopped
- 2 tablespoons olive oil
- Salt and pepper to taste

Instructions:
1. In a large mixing bowl, combine the drained and rinsed garbanzo beans, diced cucumber, finely chopped red onion, and chopped fresh parsley.
2. Drizzle the olive oil over the salad mixture. Season with salt and pepper to taste. Toss everything together until the salad ingredients are evenly coated with the olive oil and seasoning.
3. Let the salad sit for about 5 minutes to allow the flavors to meld together. This step can enhance the overall taste of the salad.
4. Serve the salad chilled or at room temperature. It can be served as a standalone dish or as a side to complement a main course.

Macronutrients:
- **Kcal:** 180
- **Carbs:** 24g
- **Protein:** 6g
- **Fat:** 8g
- **Potassium:** 290mg
- **Calcium:** 40mg
- **Magnesium:** 48mg

Ingredient Variation Tip: For an added tangy flavor, you can include a tablespoon of lemon juice or vinegar to the salad dressing.

Grilled Lemon Herb Chicken

Preparation Time: 10 minutes
Cooking Time: 10 minutes
Ingredients:
- 4 chicken breasts, boneless and skinless
- 2 lemons, juiced and zested
- 2 tablespoons olive oil
- 1 tablespoon mixed dried herbs (such as oregano, thyme, and rosemary)
- Salt and pepper to taste

Instructions:
1. In a small bowl, whisk together lemon juice, lemon zest, olive oil, mixed dried herbs, salt, and pepper to create the marinade.
2. Place the chicken breasts in a shallow dish or a resealable plastic bag. Pour the marinade over the chicken, ensuring each piece is well-coated. Marinate in the refrigerator for at least 30 minutes, or up to 2 hours for more flavor.
3. Preheat the grill to medium-high heat. Remove the chicken from the marinade, letting the excess drip off. Grill the chicken for 5 minutes on each side, or until fully cooked through and the internal temperature reaches 165°F (74°C).
4. Let the chicken rest for a few minutes before slicing and serving.

Macronutrients:
- **Kcal:** 220
- **Carbs:** 3g
- **Protein:** 26g
- **Fat:** 11g
- **Potassium:** 370mg
- **Calcium:** 20mg
- **Magnesium:** 30mg

Ingredient Variation Tip: For a citrusy twist, add a tablespoon of orange juice to the marinade.

Hummus and Veggie Wrap

Preparation Time: 5 minutes

Cooking Time: 0 minutes

Ingredients:
- 2 whole grain tortillas
- 1/2 cup hummus
- 1 cup mixed greens (spinach, arugula, or lettuce)
- 1/2 cucumber, thinly sliced
- 1/2 bell pepper, thinly sliced

Instructions:
1. Lay out the whole grain tortillas on a flat surface. Spread a quarter cup of hummus evenly over each tortilla, leaving a small border around the edge.
2. Distribute the mixed greens across the center of each tortilla on top of the hummus.
3. Arrange the cucumber and bell pepper slices evenly over the greens.
4. Carefully roll up the tortillas tightly, starting from one edge and working your way to the other. Slice each wrap in half diagonally and serve immediately.

Macronutrients:
- **Kcal:** 250
- **Carbs:** 35g
- **Protein:** 8g
- **Fat:** 9g
- **Potassium:** 297mg
- **Calcium:** 75mg
- **Magnesium:** 30mg

Ingredient Variation Tip: For a gluten-free option, substitute whole grain tortillas with gluten-free tortillas. To add more protein, include slices of grilled chicken or turkey breast.

Italian Tuna Salad

Preparation Time: 10 minutes

Cooking Time: 0 minutes

Ingredients:
- 2 cans (5 ounces each) tuna in water, drained
- 1/4 cup red onion, finely chopped
- 1/4 cup black olives, sliced
- 2 tablespoons extra virgin olive oil
- 2 tablespoons lemon juice
- Salt and pepper to taste

Instructions:
1. In a large bowl, combine the drained tuna, finely chopped red onion, and sliced black olives.
2. Drizzle the extra virgin olive oil and lemon juice over the tuna mixture. Gently toss to ensure all ingredients are well coated.
3. Season with salt and pepper to taste. Mix again lightly to distribute the seasoning evenly.
4. Serve the salad chilled or at room temperature, as preferred.

Macronutrients:
- **Kcal:** 220
- **Carbs:** 2g
- **Protein:** 25g
- **Fat:** 12g
- **Potassium:** 210mg
- **Calcium:** 30mg
- **Magnesium:** 35mg

Ingredient Variation Tip: For a Mediterranean twist, add a handful of chopped fresh parsley or basil to the salad. This not only adds a burst of flavor but also enhances the nutritional value.

Kale and Quinoa Salad

Preparation Time: 10 minutes
Cooking Time: 15 minutes
Ingredients:
- 1 cup quinoa
- 2 cups water
- 2 cups kale, stems removed and leaves chopped
- 1/4 cup dried cranberries
- 1/4 cup sliced almonds

Instructions:
1. Rinse the quinoa under cold water until the water runs clear. In a medium saucepan, bring 2 cups of water to a boil. Add the quinoa, reduce heat to low, cover, and simmer for 15 minutes, or until all the water is absorbed. Remove from heat and let it stand covered for 5 minutes. Fluff with a fork.
2. While the quinoa is cooking, steam the kale for about 5 minutes until it is slightly wilted but still vibrant green.
3. In a large bowl, combine the cooked quinoa, steamed kale, dried cranberries, and sliced almonds. Toss everything together until well mixed.
4. Serve the salad warm or at room temperature. If desired, drizzle with a dressing of your choice (not included in the ingredient count).

Macronutrients:
- **Kcal:** 320
- **Carbs:** 55g
- **Protein:** 12g
- **Fat:** 7g
- **Potassium:** 518mg
- **Calcium:** 95mg
- **Magnesium:** 150mg

Ingredient Variation Tip: Consider drizzling the salad with a lemon-tahini dressing. Simply whisk together 2 tbs of tahini, 1 tbs of lemon juice, 2 tbs of maple syrup, and 2 to 4 tbs of water.

Lemon Garlic Shrimp

Preparation Time: 5 minutes

Cooking Time: 10 minutes

Ingredients:
- 1 lb large shrimp, peeled and deveined
- 3 cloves garlic, minced
- 2 tablespoons olive oil
- Juice of 1 lemon
- Salt and pepper to taste

Instructions:
1. In a large skillet, heat the olive oil over medium heat. Add the minced garlic and sauté for about 1 minute, or until fragrant but not browned.
2. Add the shrimp to the skillet in a single layer. Season with salt and pepper. Cook for 2-3 minutes on one side, until they start to turn pink.
3. Flip the shrimp and cook for an additional 2-3 minutes, or until fully pink and cooked through.
4. Squeeze the lemon juice over the cooked shrimp and stir to combine. Serve immediately.

Macronutrients:
- **Kcal:** 240
- **Carbs:** 2g
- **Protein:** 24g
- **Fat:** 14g
- **Potassium:** 220mg
- **Calcium:** 70mg
- **Magnesium:** 30mg

Ingredient Variation Tip: For a spicy kick, add a pinch of red pepper flakes with the garlic. To make this dish more filling, serve over a bed of cooked quinoa or whole grain pasta.

Mediterranean Chickpea Salad

Preparation Time: 10 minutes

Cooking Time: 0 minutes

Ingredients:
- 1 can (15 oz) chickpeas, rinsed and drained
- 1 large cucumber, diced
- 1/2 red onion, finely chopped
- 1/4 cup fresh parsley, chopped
- 2 tablespoons olive oil
- Juice of 1 lemon
- Salt and pepper to taste

Instructions:
1. In a large mixing bowl, combine the rinsed and drained chickpeas, diced cucumber, finely chopped red onion, and chopped fresh parsley.
2. Drizzle the olive oil and lemon juice over the salad. Season with salt and pepper to taste.
3. Toss all the ingredients together until everything is evenly coated with the dressing.
4. Let the salad sit for about 5 minutes to allow the flavors to meld together before serving.

Macronutrients:
- **Kcal:** 180
- **Carbs:** 24g
- **Protein:** 6g
- **Fat:** 8g
- **Potassium:** 290mg
- **Calcium:** 50mg
- **Magnesium:** 48mg

Ingredient Variation Tip: For an extra protein boost, add crumbled feta cheese or sliced Kalamata olives. This will not only enhance the flavor but also increase the nutritional value of the salad.

Orzo and Spinach Salad

Preparation Time: 10 minutes

Cooking Time: 10 minutes

Ingredients:
- 1 cup orzo pasta
- 2 cups fresh spinach, roughly chopped
- 1/4 cup feta cheese, crumbled
- 2 tablespoons olive oil
- Salt and pepper to taste

Instructions:
1. Cook the orzo according to package instructions in a large pot of salted boiling water until al dente, about 9 minutes. Drain and rinse under cold water to stop the cooking process.
2. In a large mixing bowl, combine the cooked orzo, chopped spinach, and crumbled feta cheese. Drizzle with olive oil and season with salt and pepper to taste. Toss everything together until well mixed.
3. Let the salad sit for about 5 minutes to allow the spinach to slightly wilt and the flavors to meld together.
4. Serve chilled or at room temperature for the best flavor.

Macronutrients:
- **Kcal:** 320
- **Carbs:** 45g
- **Protein:** 10g
- **Fat:** 12g
- **Potassium:** 240mg
- **Calcium:** 150mg
- **Magnesium:** 50mg

Ingredient Variation Tip: For a protein boost, add grilled chicken or chickpeas. For a gluten-free version, substitute orzo with quinoa.

Pesto Zucchini Noodles

Preparation Time: 10 minutes

Cooking Time: 5 minutes

Ingredients:
- 2 medium zucchinis, spiralized
- 1/4 cup pesto sauce
- 1 tablespoon olive oil
- 1/4 cup grated Parmesan cheese
- Salt and pepper to taste

Instructions:
1. Heat the olive oil in a large skillet over medium heat. Add the spiralized zucchini noodles (zoodles) to the skillet, and sauté for 2-3 minutes, or until just tender. Season with salt and pepper to taste.
2. Reduce the heat to low and add the pesto sauce to the zoodles. Toss gently to coat the zoodles evenly with the pesto.
3. Cook for an additional 2 minutes, stirring occasionally, until the zoodles are heated through and fully coated with the pesto.
4. Serve the pesto zucchini noodles hot, sprinkled with grated Parmesan cheese on top.

Macronutrients:
- **Kcal:** 220
- **Carbs:** 6g
- **Protein:** 7g
- **Fat:** 18g
- **Potassium:** 512mg
- **Calcium:** 130mg
- **Magnesium:** 24mg

Ingredient Variation Tip: For a protein boost, add grilled chicken strips or shrimp to the zoodles. For a vegan option, use a dairy-free pesto and substitute the Parmesan cheese with nutritional yeast.

Quinoa and Black Bean Salad

Preparation Time: 10 minutes

Cooking Time: 0 minutes

Ingredients:
- 1 cup cooked quinoa
- 1 can (15 ounces) black beans, rinsed and drained
- 1 large tomato, diced
- 1/4 cup chopped fresh cilantro
- Juice of 1 lime

Instructions:
1. In a large bowl, combine the cooked quinoa, black beans, and diced tomato.
2. Add the chopped fresh cilantro to the bowl and pour the lime juice over the salad. Toss everything together until well mixed.
3. Taste the salad and adjust the seasoning with salt and pepper if necessary.
4. Chill the salad in the refrigerator for at least 10 minutes before serving to allow the flavors to meld together.

Macronutrients:
- **Kcal:** 220
- **Carbs:** 40g
- **Protein:** 11g
- **Fat:** 2g
- **Potassium:** 600mg
- **Calcium:** 50mg
- **Magnesium:** 70mg

Ingredient Variation Tip: For an extra crunch, add 1/4 cup of red onion finely chopped or a bell pepper diced. To enhance the protein content, include a diced grilled chicken breast or tofu cubes.

Roasted Red Pepper Hummus Wrap

Preparation Time: 5 minutes
Cooking Time: 0 minutes
Ingredients:
- 2 whole grain tortillas
- 1/2 cup roasted red pepper hummus
- 1 cup baby spinach leaves
- 1/2 cup jarred roasted red peppers, sliced
- 1/4 cup crumbled feta cheese

Instructions:
1. Lay out the whole grain tortillas on a clean, flat surface. Spread a quarter cup of roasted red pepper hummus evenly over each tortilla, leaving a small border around the edge.
2. Distribute the baby spinach leaves across the center of each tortilla on top of the hummus.
3. Arrange the sliced roasted red peppers evenly over the spinach. Sprinkle the crumbled feta cheese on top of the roasted red peppers.
4. Carefully roll up the tortillas tightly, starting from one edge and working your way to the other. Slice each wrap in half diagonally and serve immediately.

Macronutrients:
- **Kcal:** 260
- **Carbs:** 35g
- **Protein:** 10g
- **Fat:** 9g
- **Potassium:** 297mg
- **Calcium:** 100mg
- **Magnesium:** 30mg

Ingredient Variation Tip: For a gluten-free option, substitute whole grain tortillas with gluten-free tortillas. To add a protein boost, include slices of grilled chicken or turkey breast inside the wrap.

Spinach and Feta Stuffed Peppers

Preparation Time: 10 minutes

Cooking Time: 15 minutes

Ingredients:
- 4 bell peppers, halved and seeded
- 1 cup cooked spinach
- 1/2 cup crumbled feta cheese
- 1/4 cup cooked quinoa
- Salt and pepper to taste

Instructions:
1. Preheat the oven to 375°F (190°C). Arrange the bell pepper halves on a baking sheet, cut-side up.
2. In a mixing bowl, combine the cooked spinach, crumbled feta cheese, cooked quinoa, and season with salt and pepper. Mix well.
3. Spoon the spinach and feta mixture evenly into each bell pepper half.
4. Bake in the preheated oven for 15 minutes, or until the peppers are tender and the filling is heated through.

Macronutrients:
- **Kcal:** 160
- **Carbs:** 18g
- **Protein:** 7g
- **Fat:** 7g
- **Potassium:** 349mg
- **Calcium:** 150mg
- **Magnesium:** 55mg

Ingredient Variation Tip: For a protein boost, add diced grilled chicken or tofu to the spinach and feta mixture. This not only increases the protein content but also adds a savory flavor that complements the sweetness of the bell peppers.

Tomato and Cucumber Salad

Preparation Time: 10 minutes

Cooking Time: 0 minutes

Ingredients:
- 2 large cucumbers, thinly sliced
- 3 ripe tomatoes, diced
- 1/4 cup red onion, thinly sliced
- 2 tablespoons extra virgin olive oil
- Salt and pepper to taste

Instructions:
1. In a large mixing bowl, combine the thinly sliced cucumbers, diced tomatoes, and thinly sliced red onion.
2. Drizzle the vegetables with the extra virgin olive oil. Gently toss the salad to ensure all the ingredients are well coated.
3. Season the salad with salt and pepper to taste. Toss again to evenly distribute the seasoning.
4. Serve the salad immediately, or let it chill in the refrigerator for about 15 minutes to enhance the flavors.

Macronutrients:
- **Kcal:** 120
- **Carbs:** 10g
- **Protein:** 2g
- **Fat:** 9g
- **Potassium:** 360mg
- **Calcium:** 30mg
- **Magnesium:** 24mg

Ingredient Variation Tip: For an added Mediterranean flair, sprinkle some crumbled feta cheese and olives over the salad before serving. This not only introduces a new layer of flavor but also increases the protein content of the dish.

Tuna and White Bean Salad

Preparation Time: 5 minutes

Cooking Time: 0 minutes

Ingredients:
- 1 can (15 ounces) white beans, rinsed and drained
- 1 can (5 ounces) tuna in water, drained
- 1 small red onion, finely chopped
- 2 tablespoons extra virgin olive oil
- Juice of 1 lemon

Instructions:
1. In a large bowl, combine the rinsed and drained white beans and tuna.
2. Add the finely chopped red onion to the bowl.
3. Drizzle the extra virgin olive oil and squeeze the lemon juice over the salad. Gently toss to combine all the ingredients evenly.
4. Season with salt and pepper to taste, and serve immediately or chill in the refrigerator before serving.

Macronutrients:
- **Kcal:** 320
- **Carbs:** 38g
- **Protein:** 22g
- **Fat:** 9g
- **Potassium:** 800mg
- **Calcium:** 120mg
- **Magnesium:** 80mg

Ingredient Variation Tip: For an added crunch and a pop of color, include a diced red bell pepper or cucumber. This not only enhances the texture but also increases the nutritional value of the salad.

Veggie and Feta Stuffed Pita

Preparation Time: 10 minutes

Cooking Time: 5 minutes

Ingredients:
- 2 whole wheat pita breads
- 1 cup mixed vegetables (bell peppers, onions, and spinach), chopped
- 1/2 cup crumbled feta cheese
- 1 tablespoon olive oil
- Salt and pepper to taste

Instructions:
1. Heat the olive oil in a skillet over medium heat. Add the chopped vegetables and sauté until they are soft, about 3-4 minutes. Season with salt and pepper to taste.
2. Cut the pita breads in half to make pockets. Distribute the sautéed vegetables evenly among the pita pockets.
3. Sprinkle the crumbled feta cheese into the pockets with the vegetables.
4. Serve the stuffed pitas warm, or if preferred, lightly toast them in a pan for 1-2 minutes on each side to add a bit of crunch.

Macronutrients:
- **Kcal:** 320
- **Carbs:** 45g
- **Protein:** 12g
- **Fat:** 12g
- **Potassium:** 200mg
- **Calcium:** 150mg
- **Magnesium:** 30mg

Ingredient Variation Tip: For a gluten-free option, use gluten-free pita bread. To add a protein boost, include slices of grilled chicken or turkey breast inside the pita along with the vegetables and feta.

White Bean and Kale Soup

Preparation Time: 5 minutes
Cooking Time: 15 minutes
Ingredients:
- 1 can (15 oz) white beans, rinsed and drained
- 4 cups low-sodium vegetable broth
- 2 cups kale, chopped
- 1 teaspoon olive oil
- Salt and pepper to taste
Instructions:
1. Heat the olive oil in a large pot over medium heat. Add the kale and sauté for 2-3 minutes, until it starts to wilt.
2. Add the white beans and vegetable broth to the pot. Season with salt and pepper to taste. Bring the mixture to a boil.
3. Once boiling, reduce the heat to low and simmer for 10 minutes, allowing the flavors to meld together.
4. After 10 minutes, use an immersion blender to partially blend the soup, leaving some beans whole for texture. If you don't have an immersion blender, carefully transfer about half of the soup to a blender, blend until smooth, and then mix it back into the pot.
Macronutrients:
- **Kcal:** 180
- **Carbs:** 30g
- **Protein:** 10g
- **Fat:** 3g
- **Potassium:** 600mg
- **Calcium:** 100mg
- **Magnesium:** 80mg
Ingredient Variation Tip: For a heartier version, add diced carrots and celery in with the kale. This not only adds additional flavors and textures but also increases the nutritional value of the soup.

Zesty Lemon Chicken

Preparation Time: 10 minutes
Cooking Time: 10 minutes
Ingredients:
- 4 boneless, skinless chicken breasts
- 2 lemons, juiced and zested
- 2 tablespoons olive oil
- 1 teaspoon dried oregano
- Salt and pepper to taste

Instructions:
1. In a large bowl, whisk together lemon juice, lemon zest, olive oil, dried oregano, salt, and pepper. Add the chicken breasts, ensuring they are fully coated in the marinade. Let them sit for at least 5 minutes to absorb the flavors.
2. Heat a grill pan or skillet over medium-high heat. Once hot, add the chicken breasts. Cook for 5 minutes on each side, or until the chicken is thoroughly cooked and has internal temperature of 165°F (74°C).
3. Remove the chicken from the heat and let it rest for a few minutes before slicing. This helps retain the juices and flavors.
4. Serve the sliced chicken garnished with additional lemon zest or fresh oregano if desired.

Macronutrients:
- **Kcal:** 220
- **Carbs:** 0g
- **Protein:** 26g
- **Fat:** 12g
- **Potassium:** 370mg
- **Calcium:** 20mg
- **Magnesium:** 30mg

Ingredient Variation Tip: For a slightly sweeter version, add a tablespoon of honey to the marinade. This will caramelize nicely when grilled, offering a delightful contrast to the zesty lemon.

Zucchini and Tomato Bake

Preparation Time: 10 minutes

Cooking Time: 15 minutes

Ingredients:
- 2 medium zucchinis, sliced
- 3 large tomatoes, sliced
- 1/4 cup fresh basil leaves, chopped
- 2 tablespoons olive oil
- Salt and pepper to taste

Instructions:
1. Preheat the oven to 375°F (190°C). Lightly grease a baking dish with 1 tablespoon of olive oil.
2. Arrange the sliced zucchinis and tomatoes in the baking dish, alternating them and overlapping slightly for a layered effect. Sprinkle the chopped basil over the top. Season with salt and pepper to taste.
3. Drizzle the remaining tablespoon of olive oil evenly over the vegetables.
4. Bake in the preheated oven for 15 minutes, or until the vegetables are tender and the top is slightly golden.

Macronutrients:
- **Kcal:** 120
- **Carbs:** 10g
- **Protein:** 2g
- **Fat:** 9g
- **Potassium:** 510mg
- **Calcium:** 30mg
- **Magnesium:** 24mg

Ingredient Variation Tip: For added flavor, sprinkle a thin layer of grated Parmesan or mozzarella cheese over the top before baking. This will introduce a delightful cheesy crust without compromising the dish's healthful profile.

Zucchini Noodles with Pesto

Preparation Time: 10 minutes

Cooking Time: 5 minutes

Ingredients:
- 2 medium zucchinis
- 1/4 cup prepared pesto sauce
- 1 tablespoon olive oil
- 1/4 cup grated Parmesan cheese
- Salt and pepper to taste

Instructions:
1. Use a spiralizer to turn the zucchinis into noodles. If you don't have a spiralizer, use a vegetable peeler to create long, thin strips.
2. Heat the olive oil in a large skillet over medium heat. Add the zucchini noodles (zoodles) and sauté for 2-3 minutes, just until tender. Season with salt and pepper to taste.
3. Remove the skillet from heat and stir in the pesto sauce until the zoodles are evenly coated.
4. Serve the zoodles topped with grated Parmesan cheese.

Macronutrients:
- **Kcal:** 220
- **Carbs:** 6g
- **Protein:** 7g
- **Fat:** 18g
- **Potassium:** 512mg
- **Calcium:** 190mg
- **Magnesium:** 58mg

Ingredient Variation Tip: For a protein boost, add grilled chicken or shrimp to the dish. For a vegan option, use a dairy-free pesto sauce and substitute nutritional yeast for the Parmesan cheese.

Dinner Recipes

Arugula and Parmesan Salad

Preparation Time: 5 minutes

Cooking Time: 0 minutes

Ingredients:
- 4 cups arugula
- 1/2 cup shaved Parmesan cheese
- 2 tablespoons extra virgin olive oil
- 1 tablespoon lemon juice
- Salt and pepper to taste

Instructions:
1. In a large salad bowl, combine the arugula and shaved Parmesan cheese.
2. In a small bowl, whisk together the extra virgin olive oil and lemon juice. Season with salt and pepper to taste.
3. Drizzle the dressing over the arugula and Parmesan cheese. Toss gently to ensure the salad is evenly coated.
4. Serve immediately, adjusting salt and pepper as needed.

Macronutrients:
- **Kcal:** 150
- **Carbs:** 2g
- **Protein:** 7g
- **Fat:** 13g
- **Potassium:** 210mg
- **Calcium:** 220mg
- **Magnesium:** 30mg

Ingredient Variation Tip: For a crunchy texture, add a handful of toasted pine nuts or walnuts to the salad before serving.

Baked Cod with Lemon

Preparation Time: 5 minutes

Cooking Time: 15 minutes

Ingredients:
- 4 cod fillets (6 ounces each)
- 2 lemons, 1 sliced and 1 juiced
- 2 tablespoons olive oil
- Salt and pepper to taste
- Fresh parsley for garnish (optional)

Instructions:
1. Preheat the oven to 400°F (200°C). Line a baking sheet with parchment paper for easy cleanup.
2. Place the cod fillets on the prepared baking sheet. Drizzle with olive oil and lemon juice. Season with salt and pepper. Top each fillet with a couple of lemon slices.
3. Bake in the preheated oven for about 15 minutes, or until the fish flakes easily with a fork.
4. Garnish with fresh parsley before serving, if desired.

Macronutrients:
- **Kcal:** 200
- **Carbs:** 0g
- **Protein:** 31g
- **Fat:** 9g
- **Potassium:** 620mg
- **Calcium:** 20mg
- **Magnesium:** 50mg

Ingredient Variation Tip: For an herby twist, sprinkle dried thyme or dill over the cod before baking. This will add a fragrant aroma and a burst of flavor to the dish.

Broccoli and Feta Pasta

Preparation Time: 10 minutes

Cooking Time: 10 minutes

Ingredients:
- 8 oz whole wheat pasta
- 2 cups broccoli florets
- 1/2 cup crumbled feta cheese
- 2 tablespoons olive oil
- Salt and pepper to taste

Instructions:
1. Bring a large pot of salted water to a boil. Add the pasta and cook according to package instructions until al dente. In the last 3 minutes of cooking, add the broccoli florets to the pot. Drain the pasta and broccoli, reserving 1/4 cup of the pasta water.
2. Return the pasta and broccoli to the pot. Add the crumbled feta cheese and olive oil. Toss everything together until the pasta is evenly coated, adding a bit of the reserved pasta water if needed to help the cheese coat the pasta.
3. Season with salt and pepper to taste, and give everything a final toss.
4. Serve immediately, with additional feta cheese sprinkled on top if desired.

Macronutrients:
- **Kcal:** 420
- **Carbs:** 56g
- **Protein:** 16g
- **Fat:** 16g
- **Potassium:** 303mg
- **Calcium:** 200mg
- **Magnesium:** 60mg

Ingredient Variation Tip: For a gluten-free version, substitute whole wheat pasta with your favorite gluten-free pasta. To add a protein boost, include grilled chicken or chickpeas.

Cauliflower Rice Stir-Fry

Preparation Time: 5 minutes
Cooking Time: 10 minutes
Ingredients:
- 1 head of cauliflower, grated into rice-sized pieces
- 1 tablespoon olive oil
- 1/2 cup diced onions
- 1 cup mixed vegetables (carrots, peas, and corn)
- Salt and pepper to taste

Instructions:
1. Heat the olive oil in a large skillet over medium heat. Add the diced onions and sauté until they become translucent, about 2-3 minutes.
2. Add the grated cauliflower to the skillet, stirring to combine with the onions. Cook for about 5 minutes, or until the cauliflower starts to become tender.
3. Stir in the mixed vegetables, and continue to cook for another 5 minutes, or until the vegetables are heated through and the cauliflower is tender but not mushy. Season with salt and pepper to taste.
4. Serve hot as a side dish or a light main course.

Macronutrients:
- **Kcal:** 120
- **Carbs:** 14g
- **Protein:** 4g
- **Fat:** 7g
- **Potassium:** 430mg
- **Calcium:** 40mg
- **Magnesium:** 30mg

Ingredient Variation Tip: For a protein boost, add cooked, diced chicken or tofu to the stir-fry. This not only increases the protein content but also makes the dish more filling.

Chicken and Asparagus Stir-Fry

Preparation Time: 10 minutes
Cooking Time: 10 minutes
Ingredients:
- 1 lb chicken breast, thinly sliced
- 1 lb asparagus, ends trimmed and cut into 2-inch pieces
- 2 tablespoons olive oil
- Salt and pepper to taste
- 2 cloves garlic, minced

Instructions:
1. Heat 1 tablespoon of olive oil in a large skillet over medium-high heat. Season the chicken slices with salt and pepper, then add them to the skillet. Cook for 5-6 minutes, or until the chicken is golden brown and cooked through. Remove the chicken from the skillet and set aside.
2. In the same skillet, add the remaining tablespoon of olive oil and the minced garlic. Sauté for 1 minute until fragrant.
3. Add the asparagus to the skillet, season with salt and pepper, and cook for 3-4 minutes, or until tender-crisp.
4. Return the chicken to the skillet, stir to combine with the asparagus, and cook for an additional 1-2 minutes until everything is heated through.

Macronutrients:
- **Kcal:** 220
- **Carbs:** 5g
- **Protein:** 26g
- **Fat:** 11g
- **Potassium:** 400mg
- **Calcium:** 30mg
- **Magnesium:** 20mg

Ingredient Variation Tip: For a zesty flavor, add the zest of one lemon to the skillet when sautéing the garlic. This will add a fresh and tangy taste to the stir-fry.

Chicken and Broccoli Alfredo

Preparation Time: 10 minutes
Cooking Time: 10 minutes
Ingredients:
- 2 cups broccoli florets
- 8 oz chicken breast, cut into bite-sized pieces
- 1 cup whole wheat pasta, cooked according to package instructions
- 1/2 cup low-fat Alfredo sauce
- 1 tablespoon olive oil.

Instructions:
1. Heat the olive oil in a large skillet over medium heat. Add the chicken pieces and cook until they are golden brown and cooked through, about 5-7 minutes. Remove the chicken from the skillet and set aside.
2. In the same skillet, add the broccoli florets and sauté until they are tender but still crisp, about 3-4 minutes. You may add a splash of water to help steam the broccoli.
3. Return the cooked chicken to the skillet with the broccoli. Pour the Alfredo sauce over the chicken and broccoli, stirring to combine. Cook for an additional 2-3 minutes, or until everything is heated through.
4. Serve the chicken and broccoli Alfredo over the cooked whole wheat pasta.

Macronutrients:
- **Kcal:** 450
- **Carbs:** 45g
- **Protein:** 35g
- **Fat:** 15g
- **Potassium:** 500mg
- **Calcium:** 150mg
- **Magnesium:** 50mg

Ingredient Variation Tip: For a vegetarian version, substitute the chicken with white beans or chickpeas.

Chicken and Zucchini Skewers

Preparation Time: 10 minutes

Cooking Time: 10 minutes

Ingredients:
- 1 lb chicken breast, cut into 1-inch cubes
- 2 medium zucchinis, cut into 1-inch slices
- 2 tablespoons olive oil
- Salt and pepper to taste
- Wooden or metal skewers

Instructions:
1. Preheat the grill to medium-high heat. If using wooden skewers, soak them in water for at least 20 minutes to prevent burning.
2. Thread the chicken and zucchini slices alternately onto the skewers. Brush them with olive oil and season with salt and pepper.
3. Place the skewers on the grill. Cook for about 5 minutes on each side or until the chicken is thoroughly cooked and the zucchini is tender.
4. Remove from the grill and let rest for a couple of minutes before serving.

Macronutrients:
- **Kcal:** 220
- **Carbs:** 4g
- **Protein:** 26g
- **Fat:** 11g
- **Potassium:** 500mg
- **Calcium:** 20mg
- **Magnesium:** 30mg

Ingredient Variation Tip: For a vegetarian option, substitute chicken with firm tofu or halloumi cheese. Ensure to press the tofu to remove excess water before marinating.

Chicken Caprese

Preparation Time: 10 minutes

Cooking Time: 10 minutes

Ingredients:
- 2 boneless, skinless chicken breasts
- 2 large tomatoes, sliced
- 4 slices fresh mozzarella cheese
- 1/4 cup fresh basil leaves
- 2 tablespoons balsamic glaze
- Salt and pepper to taste

Instructions:
1. Season the chicken breasts with salt and pepper. Grill over medium heat for 5 minutes on each side or until the chicken is fully cooked through. Remove from the grill and let it rest for a few minutes.
2. On a serving plate, layer the sliced tomatoes and mozzarella cheese on top of the grilled chicken breasts.
3. Drizzle the balsamic glaze over the chicken, tomatoes, and mozzarella. Garnish with fresh basil leaves.
4. Serve immediately while the chicken is warm and the cheese is slightly melted.

Macronutrients:
- **Kcal:** 320
- **Carbs:** 8g
- **Protein:** 28g
- **Fat:** 18g
- **Potassium:** 410mg
- **Calcium:** 220mg
- **Magnesium:** 30mg

Ingredient Variation Tip: For a lighter version, substitute the mozzarella with a low-fat cheese option. To add a crunchy texture, include a layer of fresh arugula or spinach leaves between the chicken and the tomatoes.

Chicken Pesto Pasta

Preparation Time: 10 minutes

Cooking Time: 10 minutes

Ingredients:
- 8 oz whole wheat pasta
- 1/2 cup prepared pesto sauce
- 1 cup cooked chicken breast, diced
- 1/4 cup grated Parmesan cheese
- Salt and pepper to taste

Instructions:
1. Cook the pasta according to package instructions in a large pot of salted boiling water until al dente, about 8-10 minutes. Drain and return to the pot.
2. Add the prepared pesto sauce and diced chicken breast to the pot with the cooked pasta. Stir over low heat until the pasta is evenly coated and the chicken is heated through, about 2 minutes.
3. Season with salt and pepper to taste.
4. Serve the pasta in bowls, sprinkled with grated Parmesan cheese on top.

Macronutrients:
- **Kcal:** 450
- **Carbs:** 56g
- **Protein:** 32g
- **Fat:** 14g
- **Potassium:** 300mg
- **Calcium:** 150mg
- **Magnesium:** 60mg

Ingredient Variation Tip: For a vegetarian version, substitute the chicken with roasted vegetables such as zucchini, bell peppers, and cherry tomatoes. This not only adds a variety of textures and flavors but also enhances the dish's nutritional profile.

Garlic Shrimp and Broccoli

Preparation Time: 5 minutes

Cooking Time: 10 minutes

Ingredients:
- 1 lb large shrimp, peeled and deveined
- 2 cups broccoli florets
- 3 cloves garlic, minced
- 2 tablespoons olive oil
- Salt and pepper to taste

Instructions:
1. Heat the olive oil in a large skillet over medium heat. Add the minced garlic and sauté for about 1 minute, or until fragrant but not browned.
2. Add the broccoli florets to the skillet, season with salt and pepper, and sauté for 3-4 minutes, or until they start to become tender.
3. Add the shrimp to the skillet with the broccoli and cook for 2-3 minutes on one side, until they start to turn pink.
4. Flip the shrimp and cook for an additional 2-3 minutes, or until fully pink and cooked through. Serve immediately.

Macronutrients:
- **Kcal:** 240
- **Carbs:** 6g
- **Protein:** 24g
- **Fat:** 14g
- **Potassium:** 330mg
- **Calcium:** 120mg
- **Magnesium:** 30mg

Ingredient Variation Tip: For a spicy kick, add a pinch of red pepper flakes with the garlic. To make this dish more filling, serve over a bed of cooked quinoa or whole grain pasta.

Grilled Chicken with Avocado Salsa

Preparation Time: 10 minutes
Cooking Time: 10 minutes
Ingredients:
- 4 chicken breasts, boneless and skinless
- 2 avocados, diced
- 1/4 cup fresh cilantro, chopped
- Juice of 1 lime
- Salt and pepper to taste

Instructions:
1. Preheat the grill to medium-high heat. Season the chicken breasts with salt and pepper, then place them on the grill. Cook for 5 minutes on each side, or until the chicken is thoroughly cooked and has internal temperature of 165°F (74°C).
2. In a medium bowl, combine the diced avocados, chopped cilantro, and lime juice. Season with salt and pepper to taste, and gently mix to combine.
3. Once the chicken is cooked, remove it from the grill and let it rest for a few minutes.
4. Serve the grilled chicken topped with the avocado salsa.

Macronutrients:
- **Kcal:** 320
- **Carbs:** 9g
- **Protein:** 26g
- **Fat:** 20g
- **Potassium:** 650mg
- **Calcium:** 30mg
- **Magnesium:** 45mg

Ingredient Variation Tip: For a spicy twist, add diced jalapeños to the avocado salsa. This will introduce a kick of heat that complements the creamy texture of the avocado and the savory flavor of the grilled chicken.

Grilled Eggplant with Feta

Preparation Time: 10 minutes
Cooking Time: 15 minutes
Ingredients:
- 1 large eggplant, sliced into 1/2-inch rounds
- 2 large tomatoes, sliced
- 1/4 cup low-fat ricotta cheese
- 2 tablespoons fresh basil, chopped
- Salt and pepper to taste

Instructions:
1. Preheat a grill or grill pan over medium heat. Season the eggplant slices with salt and pepper, and grill for about 4-5 minutes on each side, or until tender and grill marks appear.
2. On a serving plate, layer a slice of grilled eggplant, then a slice of tomato, and a teaspoon of ricotta cheese. Repeat the layering process until all ingredients are used, finishing with a dollop of ricotta on top.
3. Garnish the stack with fresh basil. Serve immediately or at room temperature.
4. For a richer flavor, you can drizzle a little balsamic glaze over the top before serving.

Macronutrients:
- **Kcal:** 180
- **Carbs:** 22g
- **Protein:** 9g
- **Fat:** 8g
- **Potassium:** 676mg
- **Calcium:** 150mg
- **Magnesium:** 55mg

Ingredient Variation Tip: For a vegan version, substitute ricotta cheese with a vegan almond or cashew cheese. To add a crunchy texture, sprinkle some toasted pine nuts or walnuts on top before serving.

Lemon Herb Salmon

Preparation Time: 5 minutes

Cooking Time: 15 minutes

Ingredients:
- 4 salmon fillets (6 ounces each)
- 2 tablespoons olive oil
- 2 lemons, one juiced and one sliced
- 1 tablespoon fresh dill, chopped
- Salt and pepper to taste

Instructions:
1. Preheat the oven to 400°F (200°C). Line a baking sheet with parchment paper.
2. Place the salmon fillets on the prepared baking sheet. Drizzle with olive oil and lemon juice. Season with salt and pepper. Top each fillet with a few slices of lemon and sprinkle with chopped dill.
3. Bake in the preheated oven for 12-15 minutes, or until the salmon flakes easily with a fork.
4. Serve immediately, garnished with additional fresh dill if desired.

Macronutrients:
- **Kcal:** 280
- **Carbs:** 0g
- **Protein:** 23g
- **Fat:** 20g
- **Potassium:** 555mg
- **Calcium:** 20mg
- **Magnesium:** 30mg

Ingredient Variation Tip: For a different flavor profile, try substituting dill with fresh rosemary or thyme.

Lentil and Veggie Stew

Preparation Time: 10 minutes

Cooking Time: 15 minutes

Ingredients:
- 1 cup dried lentils, rinsed
- 4 cups low-sodium vegetable broth
- 1 cup diced carrots
- 1 cup diced celery
- 1 teaspoon dried thyme

Instructions:
1. In a large pot, combine the rinsed lentils and vegetable broth. Bring to a boil over high heat, then reduce the heat to low, cover, and simmer for 10 minutes.
2. Add the diced carrots and celery to the pot. Continue to simmer, covered, for another 5 minutes, or until the vegetables and lentils are tender.
3. Stir in the dried thyme and simmer for an additional minute, allowing the flavors to meld together.
4. Taste and adjust seasoning with salt and pepper if necessary. Serve hot.

Macronutrients:
- **Kcal:** 230
- **Carbs:** 40g
- **Protein:** 15g
- **Fat:** 1g
- **Potassium:** 710mg
- **Calcium:** 40mg
- **Magnesium:** 70mg

Ingredient Variation Tip: For a heartier stew, add a cup of diced tomatoes during the last 5 minutes of cooking. This not only adds a rich flavor and texture but also boosts the nutritional content.

Mediterranean Chicken Wrap

Preparation Time: 10 minutes

Cooking Time: 5 minutes

Ingredients:
- 2 whole wheat tortillas
- 1/2 lb cooked chicken breast, thinly sliced
- 1/4 cup hummus
- 1/2 cup mixed greens (spinach, arugula, or lettuce)
- 1/4 cup diced tomatoes

Instructions:
1. Lay out the whole wheat tortillas on a clean, flat surface. Spread a layer of hummus evenly over each tortilla.
2. Distribute the cooked chicken slices evenly on top of the hummus layer on each tortilla.
3. Add a layer of mixed greens and diced tomatoes over the chicken on each tortilla.
4. Carefully roll up the tortillas tightly, starting from one edge and working your way to the other. Slice each wrap in half diagonally and serve immediately.

Macronutrients:
- **Kcal:** 320
- **Carbs:** 35g
- **Protein:** 25g
- **Fat:** 9g
- **Potassium:** 400mg
- **Calcium:** 80mg
- **Magnesium:** 45mg

Ingredient Variation Tip: For a vegetarian version, substitute the chicken with grilled zucchini and eggplant slices. This not only makes the recipe suitable for vegetarians but also adds a different texture and flavor profile to the wrap.

Mediterranean Quinoa Bowl

Preparation Time: 10 minutes

Cooking Time: 15 minutes

Ingredients:
- 1 cup quinoa
- 2 cups vegetable broth
- 1 cup cherry tomatoes, halved
- 1/2 cup cucumber, diced
- 1/4 cup feta cheese, crumbled

Instructions:
1. Rinse the quinoa under cold water until the water runs clear. In a medium saucepan, combine the quinoa and vegetable broth. Bring to a boil, then reduce heat to low, cover, and simmer for about 15 minutes, or until the quinoa is tender and the broth has been absorbed.
2. Fluff the cooked quinoa with a fork and transfer it to a large mixing bowl. Allow it to cool for a few minutes.
3. Add the halved cherry tomatoes, diced cucumber, and crumbled feta cheese to the quinoa. Gently toss to combine.
4. Serve the Mediterranean Quinoa Bowl either warm or chilled, based on personal preference.

Macronutrients:
- **Kcal:** 320
- **Carbs:** 45g
- **Protein:** 12g
- **Fat:** 10g
- **Potassium:** 410mg
- **Calcium:** 150mg
- **Magnesium:** 60mg

Ingredient Variation Tip: For added protein, include grilled chicken or chickpeas. For a vegan version, substitute feta cheese with a vegan cheese alternative or simply omit it.

Pasta Primavera

Preparation Time: 10 minutes
Cooking Time: 10 minutes
Ingredients:
- 8 oz whole wheat spaghetti
- 1 cup cherry tomatoes, halved
- 1 cup asparagus, chopped
- 1/2 cup frozen peas
- 1/4 cup pesto sauce
- Salt and pepper to taste

Instructions:
1. Cook the whole wheat spaghetti according to package instructions in a large pot of salted boiling water until al dente. Drain and set aside, reserving 1/4 cup of the pasta water.
2. In the same pot, add the cherry tomatoes, asparagus, and frozen peas. Cook over medium heat for about 5 minutes, or until the vegetables are tender.
3. Return the cooked spaghetti to the pot with the vegetables. Add the pesto sauce and reserved pasta water. Toss everything together until the pasta and vegetables are well coated with the pesto. Season with salt and pepper to taste.
4. Serve hot, garnished with additional grated Parmesan cheese if desired.

Macronutrients:
- **Kcal:** 320
- **Carbs:** 48g
- **Protein:** 12g
- **Fat:** 10g
- **Potassium:** 370mg
- **Calcium:** 60mg
- **Magnesium:** 75mg

Ingredient Variation Tip: For a protein boost, add grilled chicken or shrimp to the pasta. For a vegan version, use a dairy-free pesto sauce.

Roasted Brussels Sprouts with Balsamic Glaze

Preparation Time: 10 minutes

Cooking Time: 15 minutes

Ingredients:
- 1 lb Brussels sprouts, trimmed and halved
- 2 tablespoons olive oil
- Salt and pepper to taste
- 2 tablespoons balsamic glaze

Instructions:
1. Preheat your oven to 400°F (200°C). In a large bowl, toss the Brussels sprouts with olive oil, salt, and pepper until they are evenly coated.
2. Spread the Brussels sprouts on a baking sheet in a single layer, ensuring the cut sides are facing down.
3. Roast in the preheated oven for about 15 minutes, or until they are tender on the inside and crispy on the outside.
4. Drizzle the balsamic glaze over the roasted Brussels sprouts before serving.

Macronutrients:
- **Kcal:** 150
- **Carbs:** 18g
- **Protein:** 6g
- **Fat:** 7g
- **Potassium:** 441mg
- **Calcium:** 56mg
- **Magnesium:** 31mg

Ingredient Variation Tip: For a sweet and spicy twist, mix a pinch of red pepper flakes into the olive oil before tossing with the Brussels sprouts.

Roasted Cauliflower Tacos

Preparation Time: 10 minutes
Cooking Time: 15 minutes
Ingredients:
- 1 head cauliflower, cut into small florets
- 2 tablespoons olive oil
- 1 teaspoon chili powder
- 1/2 teaspoon garlic powder
- Salt and pepper to taste
- 8 small corn tortillas
- Optional toppings: diced avocado, salsa, lime wedges, and fresh cilantro

Instructions:
1. Preheat the oven to 425°F (220°C). In a large bowl, toss the cauliflower florets with olive oil, chili powder, garlic powder, salt, and pepper until well coated.
2. Spread the cauliflower in a single layer on a baking sheet. Roast in the preheated oven for 15 minutes, or until tender and slightly caramelized, stirring halfway through.
3. Warm the corn tortillas in the oven for the last few minutes of the cauliflower cooking time or heat them in a dry skillet over medium heat for about 30 seconds on each side.
4. Assemble the tacos by placing a spoonful of roasted cauliflower on each tortilla. Add optional toppings like diced avocado, salsa, lime wedges, and fresh cilantro as desired.

Macronutrients:
- **Kcal:** 150 per serving (2 tacos)
- **Carbs:** 20g
- **Protein:** 4g
- **Fat:** 7g
- **Potassium:** 430mg
- **Calcium:** 40mg
- **Magnesium:** 30mg

Ingredient Variation Tip: For a heartier meal, add black beans or shredded chicken to the tacos.

Shrimp and Avocado Salad

Preparation Time: 10 minutes

Cooking Time: 0 minutes

Ingredients:
- 1 lb cooked shrimp, peeled and deveined
- 2 ripe avocados, diced
- 1/4 cup red onion, finely chopped
- 2 tablespoons lime juice
- Salt and pepper to taste

Instructions:

1. In a large mixing bowl, combine the cooked shrimp and diced avocados.

2. Add the finely chopped red onion to the bowl.

3. Drizzle the lime juice over the mixture and season with salt and pepper to taste. Gently toss to ensure all ingredients are evenly coated.

4. Chill the salad in the refrigerator for about 5 minutes before serving to allow the flavors to meld together.

Macronutrients:
- **Kcal:** 320
- **Carbs:** 14g
- **Protein:** 25g
- **Fat:** 20g
- **Potassium:** 650mg
- **Calcium:** 150mg
- **Magnesium:** 55mg

Ingredient Variation Tip: For a spicy twist, add a diced jalapeño or a dash of chili flakes to the salad. This will add a kick that complements the creamy avocado and the succulent shrimp beautifully.

Spinach and Mushroom Quesadilla

Preparation Time: 5 minutes
Cooking Time: 10 minutes
Ingredients:
- 2 large whole wheat tortillas
- 1 cup fresh spinach, roughly chopped
- 1 cup sliced mushrooms
- 1/2 cup shredded mozzarella cheese
- 1 tablespoon olive oil
Instructions:

1. Heat the olive oil in a skillet over medium heat. Add the sliced mushrooms and sauté until they are soft and lightly browned, about 5-7 minutes. Add the spinach to the skillet in the last minute of cooking, just until wilted.

2. Lay out the whole wheat tortillas on a flat surface. Evenly distribute the sautéed mushrooms and spinach over one half of each tortilla. Sprinkle the shredded mozzarella cheese on top of the vegetables.

3. Fold the tortillas in half over the filling to create a half-moon shape. Press down gently to seal.

4. Place the quesadillas in a skillet over medium heat. Cook for about 2-3 minutes on each side, or until the tortillas are crispy and the cheese has melted. Cut into wedges and serve immediately.

Macronutrients:
- **Kcal:** 320
- **Carbs:** 35g
- **Protein:** 15g
- **Fat:** 15g
- **Potassium:** 297mg
- **Calcium:** 200mg
- **Magnesium:** 30mg

Ingredient Variation Tip: For a vegan version, substitute mozzarella cheese with a dairy-free cheese alternative. To add a protein boost, include cooked, shredded chicken or black beans inside the quesadilla before cooking.

Stuffed Bell Peppers

Preparation Time: 10 minutes

Cooking Time: 15 minutes

Ingredients:
- 4 bell peppers, halved and seeded
- 1 cup cooked quinoa
- 1/2 cup crumbled feta cheese
- 1 cup spinach, cooked and drained
- Salt and pepper to taste

Instructions:
1. Preheat the oven to 375°F (190°C). Arrange the bell pepper halves on a baking sheet, cut-side up.
2. In a mixing bowl, combine the cooked quinoa, crumbled feta cheese, and cooked spinach. Season with salt and pepper to taste. Mix well.
3. Spoon the quinoa mixture evenly into each bell pepper half.
4. Bake in the preheated oven for 15 minutes, or until the peppers are tender and the filling is heated through.

Macronutrients:
- **Kcal:** 160
- **Carbs:** 18g
- **Protein:** 7g
- **Fat:** 7g
- **Potassium:** 349mg
- **Calcium:** 150mg
- **Magnesium:** 55mg

Ingredient Variation Tip: For a protein boost, add diced grilled chicken or tofu to the quinoa mixture. This not only increases the protein content but also adds a savory flavor that complements the sweetness of the bell peppers.

Tomato Basil Chicken

Preparation Time: 10 minutes
Cooking Time: 15 minutes
Ingredients:
- 4 boneless, skinless chicken breasts
- 2 tablespoons olive oil
- 1/4 cup fresh basil leaves, finely chopped
- 2 large tomatoes, sliced
- Salt and pepper to taste
Instructions:
1. Season the chicken breasts with salt and pepper. Heat the olive oil in a large skillet over medium-high heat. Add the chicken breasts and cook for 6-7 minutes on each side, or until fully cooked through and golden brown.
2. In the last 2 minutes of cooking, add the sliced tomatoes on top of the chicken breasts, allowing them to warm through.
3. Sprinkle the finely chopped basil over the chicken and tomatoes in the skillet, letting the basil infuse its flavor for about a minute.
4. Remove from heat and serve immediately, ensuring each chicken breast is topped with tomato slices and garnished with fresh basil.
Macronutrients:
- **Kcal:** 220
- **Carbs:** 5g
- **Protein:** 26g
- **Fat:** 11g
- **Potassium:** 370mg
- **Calcium:** 20mg
- **Magnesium:** 30mg
Ingredient Variation Tip: For a cheesy twist, add a slice of mozzarella cheese on top of each chicken breast during the last 3 minutes of cooking. This will add a creamy texture and rich flavor that complements the tomato and basil beautifully.

Turkey and Spinach Meatballs

Preparation Time: 10 minutes
Cooking Time: 15 minutes
Ingredients:
- 1 lb ground turkey
- 2 cups fresh spinach, finely chopped
- 1/4 cup whole wheat breadcrumbs
- 1 large egg
- Salt and pepper to taste

Instructions:
1. In a large bowl, combine the ground turkey, finely chopped spinach, whole wheat breadcrumbs, and egg. Season with salt and pepper. Mix well until all ingredients are evenly distributed.
2. Form the mixture into small, round meatballs, about 1 inch in diameter. Place them on a plate or baking sheet.
3. Heat a non-stick skillet over medium heat. Add the meatballs to the skillet, cooking them in batches if necessary to avoid overcrowding. Cook for about 7-8 minutes on each side, or until they are browned on the outside and no longer pink in the center.
4. Serve the meatballs hot, either on their own or with a side of whole grain pasta or a fresh salad.

Macronutrients:
- **Kcal:** 220
- **Carbs:** 8g
- **Protein:** 27g
- **Fat:** 9g
- **Potassium:** 340mg
- **Calcium:** 60mg
- **Magnesium:** 30mg

Ingredient Variation Tip: For a gluten-free version, substitute whole wheat breadcrumbs with almond flour or gluten-free breadcrumbs. To add a Mediterranean twist, mix in some feta cheese and oregano with the turkey and spinach mixture before forming the meatballs.

Zucchini and Tomato Gratin

Preparation Time: 10 minutes

Cooking Time: 15 minutes

Ingredients:
- 2 medium zucchinis, sliced
- 3 large tomatoes, sliced
- 1/4 cup fresh basil leaves, chopped
- 2 tablespoons olive oil
- Salt and pepper to taste

Instructions:
1. Preheat the oven to 375°F (190°C). Lightly grease a baking dish with 1 tablespoon of olive oil.
2. Arrange the sliced zucchinis and tomatoes in the baking dish, alternating them and overlapping slightly for a layered effect. Sprinkle the chopped basil over the top. Season with salt and pepper to taste.
3. Drizzle the remaining tablespoon of olive oil evenly over the vegetables.
4. Bake in the preheated oven for 15 minutes, or until the vegetables are tender and the top is slightly golden.

Macronutrients:
- **Kcal:** 120
- **Carbs:** 10g
- **Protein:** 2g
- **Fat:** 9g
- **Potassium:** 510mg
- **Calcium:** 30mg
- **Magnesium:** 24mg

Ingredient Variation Tip: For added flavor, sprinkle a thin layer of grated Parmesan or mozzarella cheese over the top before baking. This will introduce a delightful cheesy crust without compromising the dish's healthful profile.

Snacks and Appetizers Recipes

Stuffed Mini Peppers

Preparation Time: 10 minutes
Cooking Time: 10 minutes
Ingredients:
- 12 mini bell peppers, halved and seeded
- 1 cup cooked quinoa
- 1/2 cup black beans, rinsed and drained
- 1/2 cup corn kernels
- 1/2 cup shredded cheddar cheese
- Salt and pepper to taste

Instructions:
1. Preheat the oven to 375°F (190°C). Arrange the halved mini bell peppers on a baking sheet.
2. In a bowl, mix together the cooked quinoa, black beans, corn kernels, and half of the shredded cheddar cheese. Season with salt and pepper.
3. Spoon the mixture into each bell pepper half. Sprinkle the remaining cheddar cheese on top of each stuffed pepper.
4. Bake in the preheated oven for 10 minutes, or until the peppers are tender and the cheese is melted and slightly golden.

Macronutrients:
- **Kcal:** 150
- **Carbs:** 18g
- **Protein:** 8g
- **Fat:** 5g
- **Potassium:** 320mg
- **Calcium:** 120mg
- **Magnesium:** 45mg

Ingredient Variation Tip: For a Mediterranean twist, substitute black beans with chickpeas and cheddar cheese with feta cheese. Add diced olives and a sprinkle of oregano for enhanced flavor.

Cucumber Avocado Bites

Preparation Time: 10 minutes

Cooking Time: 0 minutes

Ingredients:
- 1 large cucumber, sliced into rounds
- 1 ripe avocado, mashed
- 1/4 teaspoon salt
- 1/4 teaspoon pepper
- 1 tablespoon lime juice

Instructions:
1. In a small bowl, mix the mashed avocado with salt, pepper, and lime juice until well combined.
2. Place cucumber rounds on a serving platter.
3. Top each cucumber round with a spoonful of the avocado mixture.
4. Serve immediately or chill in the refrigerator for up to 1 hour before serving.

Macronutrients:
- **Kcal:** 50 per serving (2 bites)
- **Carbs:** 4g
- **Protein:** 1g
- **Fat:** 4g
- **Potassium:** 150mg
- **Calcium:** 10mg
- **Magnesium:** 14mg

Ingredient Variation Tip: For an extra kick, sprinkle a small amount of chili powder or paprika on top of each bite before serving.

Garlic Parmesan Zucchini Chips

Preparation Time: 10 minutes

Cooking Time: 15 minutes

Ingredients:
- 2 medium zucchinis
- 1/4 cup grated Parmesan cheese
- 1 tablespoon olive oil
- 1/2 teaspoon garlic powder
- Salt and pepper to taste

Instructions:
1. Preheat your oven to 425°F (220°C). Line a baking sheet with parchment paper.
2. Slice the zucchinis into thin rounds, about 1/8 inch thick. In a bowl, toss the zucchini slices with olive oil, garlic powder, salt, and pepper until evenly coated.
3. Arrange the zucchini slices in a single layer on the prepared baking sheet. Sprinkle the grated Parmesan cheese over the zucchini slices.
4. Bake in the preheated oven for 15 minutes, or until the zucchini is tender and the Parmesan is crispy and golden. Serve immediately.

Macronutrients:
- **Kcal:** 100
- **Carbs:** 4g
- **Protein:** 6g
- **Fat:** 7g
- **Potassium:** 340mg
- **Calcium:** 130mg
- **Magnesium:** 22mg

Ingredient Variation Tip: For a spicy twist, add a pinch of chili flakes before baking. This will add a nice heat that complements the savory Parmesan and garlic flavors.

Greek Salad Skewers

Preparation Time: 10 minutes

Cooking Time: 0 minutes

Ingredients:
- 1 pint cherry tomatoes, halved
- 1 cucumber, cut into bite-sized pieces
- 1/2 cup Kalamata olives, pitted
- 1/2 cup feta cheese, cut into small cubes
- 1/4 cup fresh basil leaves
- Wooden skewers

Instructions:
1. Start by threading a cherry tomato half onto a skewer, followed by a piece of cucumber.
2. Next, add an olive, a cube of feta cheese, and then another cherry tomato half to secure everything in place. If desired, garnish each skewer with a basil leaf for an extra burst of flavor.
3. Repeat the process until all ingredients are used up, creating a colorful array of Greek Salad Skewers.
4. Serve immediately, or chill in the refrigerator until ready to serve.

Macronutrients:
- **Kcal:** 80
- **Carbs:** 4g
- **Protein:** 2g
- **Fat:** 6g
- **Potassium:** 95mg
- **Calcium:** 60mg
- **Magnesium:** 15mg

Ingredient Variation Tip: For a twist, drizzle the skewers with a balsamic reduction or olive oil before serving. This adds a rich depth of flavor that complements the fresh ingredients beautifully.

Hummus Stuffed Cherry Tomatoes

Preparation Time: 10 minutes

Cooking Time: 0 minutes

Ingredients:
- 24 cherry tomatoes
- 1 cup hummus
- 1/4 cup pine nuts, toasted
- Fresh parsley, chopped for garnish
- Salt and pepper to taste

Instructions:
1. Slice the top off each cherry tomato and carefully scoop out the seeds and inner flesh to create a hollow space. Lightly season the inside of each tomato with salt and pepper.
2. Fill each cherry tomato with hummus using a small spoon or a piping bag for a neater finish.
3. Sprinkle the top of each hummus-filled tomato with toasted pine nuts and garnish with chopped fresh parsley.
4. Chill in the refrigerator for about 5 minutes before serving to allow the flavors to meld together.

Macronutrients:
- **Kcal:** 35 per tomato
- **Carbs:** 3g
- **Protein:** 1g
- **Fat:** 2g
- **Potassium:** 44mg
- **Calcium:** 8mg
- **Magnesium:** 6mg

Ingredient Variation Tip: For a Greek twist, mix feta cheese into the hummus before stuffing the tomatoes. This adds a creamy texture and tangy flavor that pairs well with the sweetness of the cherry tomatoes.

Mediterranean Deviled Eggs

Preparation Time: 10 minutes

Cooking Time: 0 minutes

Ingredients:
- 6 hard-boiled eggs, peeled
- 1/4 cup hummus
- 1 tablespoon olive oil
- 1 teaspoon paprika
- Salt and pepper to taste

Instructions:
1. Cut the hard-boiled eggs in half lengthwise. Gently remove the yolks and place them in a small bowl.
2. Add hummus, olive oil, paprika, salt, and pepper to the yolks. Mash and mix until smooth and well combined.
3. Spoon or pipe the hummus and yolk mixture back into the egg white halves.
4. Sprinkle a little paprika over the top for garnish before serving.

Macronutrients:
- **Kcal:** 140
- **Carbs:** 2g
- **Protein:** 8g
- **Fat:** 11g
- **Potassium:** 126mg
- **Calcium:** 30mg
- **Magnesium:** 12mg

Ingredient Variation Tip: For a spicy twist, mix a small amount of sriracha or diced jalapeño into the hummus and yolk mixture.

Pesto Stuffed Mushrooms

Preparation Time: 10 minutes

Cooking Time: 15 minutes

Ingredients:
- 12 large mushrooms, stems removed
- 1/2 cup pesto sauce
- 1/4 cup grated Parmesan cheese
- 1/4 cup breadcrumbs
- 1 tablespoon olive oil

Instructions:
1. Preheat the oven to 375°F (190°C). Arrange the mushroom caps on a baking sheet, hollow sides up.
2. Spoon pesto sauce into each mushroom cap, filling them evenly. Sprinkle grated Parmesan cheese on top of the pesto.
3. In a small bowl, mix breadcrumbs with olive oil until well combined. Sprinkle this mixture over the mushrooms, covering the pesto and cheese.
4. Bake in the preheated oven for 15 minutes, or until the mushrooms are tender and the topping is golden brown.

Macronutrients:
- **Kcal:** 150
- **Carbs:** 6g
- **Protein:** 5g
- **Fat:** 12g
- **Potassium:** 223mg
- **Calcium:** 130mg
- **Magnesium:** 22mg

Ingredient Variation Tip: For a gluten-free version, substitute breadcrumbs with almond meal or gluten-free breadcrumbs. To add a spicy kick, mix a pinch of red pepper flakes into the pesto sauce before filling the mushrooms.

Roasted Chickpeas

Preparation Time: 10 minutes

Cooking Time: 15 minutes

Ingredients:
- 1 can (15 oz) chickpeas, drained and rinsed
- 1 tablespoon olive oil
- 1/2 teaspoon salt
- 1/4 teaspoon ground cumin
- 1/4 teaspoon paprika

Instructions:
1. Preheat your oven to 400°F (200°C). Line a baking sheet with parchment paper for easy cleanup.
2. In a bowl, toss the chickpeas with olive oil, salt, cumin, and paprika until evenly coated.
3. Spread the chickpeas in a single layer on the prepared baking sheet. Bake for 15 minutes, or until the chickpeas are crispy and golden brown. Stir halfway through to ensure even cooking.
4. Remove from the oven and let cool for a few minutes before serving. They will continue to crisp up as they cool.

Macronutrients:
- **Kcal:** 210
- **Carbs:** 35g
- **Protein:** 10g
- **Fat:** 5g
- **Potassium:** 329mg
- **Calcium:** 80mg
- **Magnesium:** 48mg

Ingredient Variation Tip: For a spicy version, add a pinch of chili powder or cayenne pepper to the seasoning mix before roasting.

Spinach and Feta Stuffed Mushrooms

Preparation Time: 10 minutes

Cooking Time: 15 minutes

Ingredients:
- 12 large mushrooms, stems removed
- 1 cup spinach, finely chopped
- 1/2 cup feta cheese, crumbled
- 1 tablespoon olive oil
- Salt and pepper to taste

Instructions:
1. Preheat the oven to 375°F (190°C). Arrange the mushroom caps on a baking sheet, hollow side up.
2. In a skillet over medium heat, warm the olive oil. Add the spinach and sauté until wilted, about 2-3 minutes. Season with salt and pepper.
3. Remove from heat and let cool slightly. Stir in the crumbled feta cheese. Fill each mushroom cap with the spinach and feta mixture.
4. Bake in the preheated oven for 15 minutes, or until the mushrooms are tender and the filling is heated through.

Macronutrients:
- **Kcal:** 120
- **Carbs:** 4g
- **Protein:** 6g
- **Fat:** 9g
- **Potassium:** 300mg
- **Calcium:** 150mg
- **Magnesium:** 24mg

Ingredient Variation Tip: For a crunchy texture, sprinkle breadcrumbs on top of the stuffed mushrooms before baking.

Tomato Basil Skewers

Preparation Time: 10 minutes

Cooking Time: 0 minutes

Ingredients:
- 1 pint cherry tomatoes
- 1 bunch fresh basil leaves
- 8 oz mozzarella cheese, cut into small cubes
- 2 tablespoons extra virgin olive oil
- Salt and pepper to taste

Instructions:
1. Wash the cherry tomatoes and basil leaves. Pat dry with a paper towel to remove any excess moisture.
2. On a skewer, alternate threading a cherry tomato, a basil leaf folded in half, and a cube of mozzarella cheese. Repeat until the skewer is filled, leaving enough space at the bottom to hold.
3. Once all skewers are assembled, arrange them on a serving platter. Drizzle with extra virgin olive oil and season with salt and pepper to taste.
4. Serve immediately or refrigerate until ready to serve.

Macronutrients:
- **Kcal:** 150
- **Carbs:** 2g
- **Protein:** 8g
- **Fat:** 12g
- **Potassium:** 90mg
- **Calcium:** 200mg
- **Magnesium:** 15mg

Ingredient Variation Tip: For a tangy twist, drizzle balsamic glaze over the skewers before serving. This adds a rich, sweet, and slightly acidic flavor that complements the freshness of the tomatoes and basil beautifully.

Salads and Sides Recipes

Apple Walnut Salad

Preparation time: 10 minutes

Cooking time: 0 minutes

Ingredients:
- 2 large apples, cored and chopped
- 1/2 cup walnuts, chopped
- 1/4 cup dried cranberries
- 2 tablespoons honey
- 1/2 teaspoon cinnamon

Instructions:
1. In a large bowl, combine the chopped apples, walnuts, and dried cranberries.
2. Drizzle honey over the apple mixture and sprinkle with cinnamon. Toss everything together until the apples and nuts are well coated.
3. Let the salad sit for about 5 minutes to allow the flavors to meld together.
4. Serve chilled or at room temperature.

Macronutrients:
- **kcal:** 210
- **Carbs:** 30g
- **Protein:** 3g
- **Fat:** 10g
- **Potassium:** 170mg
- **Calcium:** 20mg
- **Magnesium:** 30mg

Ingredient Variation Tip: For a creamy texture, add a dollop of Greek yogurt on top of the salad before serving. This not only adds a tangy flavor but also increases the protein content.

Beet and Goat Cheese Salad

Preparation Time: 10 minutes

Cooking Time: 0 minutes

Ingredients:
- 2 medium beets, cooked and sliced
- 1/2 cup goat cheese, crumbled
- 1/4 cup walnuts, toasted and chopped
- 2 tablespoons balsamic vinegar
- Salt and pepper to taste

Instructions:
1. Arrange the sliced beets on a serving platter or individual plates.
2. Sprinkle the crumbled goat cheese and toasted walnuts evenly over the beets.
3. Drizzle balsamic vinegar over the salad. Season with salt and pepper to taste.
4. Serve immediately or chill in the refrigerator for about 15 minutes before serving for a refreshing touch.

Macronutrients:
- **Kcal:** 220
- **Carbs:** 13g
- **Protein:** 9g
- **Fat:** 16g
- **Potassium:** 380mg
- **Calcium:** 80mg
- **Magnesium:** 40mg

Ingredient Variation Tip: For a sweet and crunchy variation, add sliced strawberries or apples and replace walnuts with pecans.

Carrot and Chickpea Salad

Preparation time: 10 minutes

Cooking time: 0 minutes

Ingredients:
- 2 cups shredded carrots
- 1 can (15 oz) chickpeas, rinsed and drained
- 1/4 cup chopped fresh parsley
- 2 tablespoons olive oil
- Juice of 1 lemon

Instructions:
1. In a large bowl, combine the shredded carrots, rinsed and drained chickpeas, and chopped fresh parsley.
2. Drizzle the olive oil and lemon juice over the carrot and chickpea mixture. Toss well to ensure all ingredients are evenly coated.
3. Season the salad with salt and pepper to taste. Mix again to distribute the seasoning evenly.
4. Chill the salad in the refrigerator for about 10 minutes before serving to allow the flavors to meld together.

Macronutrients:
- **Kcal:** 180
- **Carbs:** 24g
- **Protein:** 6g
- **Fat:** 8g
- **Potassium:** 290mg
- **Calcium:** 60mg
- **Magnesium:** 45mg

Ingredient Variation Tip: For a sweet and crunchy twist, add a handful of raisins or chopped walnuts to the salad before chilling.

Citrus Avocado Salad

Preparation time: 10 minutes

Cooking time: 0 minutes

Ingredients:
- 2 large oranges, peeled and sectioned
- 1 ripe avocado, peeled, pitted, and sliced
- 1/4 red onion, thinly sliced
- 2 tablespoons olive oil
- Salt and pepper to taste

Instructions:
1. Arrange the orange sections and avocado slices on a serving platter.
2. Scatter the thinly sliced red onion over the top.
3. Drizzle with olive oil and season with salt and pepper to taste.
4. Serve immediately or chill in the refrigerator for up to 1 hour before serving to allow the flavors to meld together.

Macronutrients:
- **Kcal:** 250
- **Carbs:** 20g
- **Protein:** 3g
- **Fat:** 20g
- **Potassium:** 490mg
- **Calcium:** 60mg
- **Magnesium:** 30mg

Ingredient Variation Tip: For an added crunch and nutty flavor, sprinkle toasted almond slices over the salad before serving.

Fennel and Orange Salad

Preparation time: 10 minutes

Cooking time: 0 minutes

Ingredients:
- 2 medium fennel bulbs, thinly sliced
- 2 oranges, peeled and sectioned
- 2 tablespoons olive oil
- Salt and pepper to taste
- 1/4 cup sliced almonds, toasted

Instructions:
1. In a large mixing bowl, combine the thinly sliced fennel bulbs and orange sections.
2. Drizzle the olive oil over the fennel and oranges. Season with salt and pepper to taste. Toss gently to ensure the salad is evenly coated.
3. Chill the salad in the refrigerator for about 5 minutes to allow the flavors to meld together.
4. Just before serving, sprinkle the toasted sliced almonds over the top of the salad for added crunch.

Macronutrients:
- **Kcal:** 180
- **Carbs:** 18g
- **Protein:** 3g
- **Fat:** 12g
- **Potassium:** 360mg
- **Calcium:** 75mg
- **Magnesium:** 30mg

Ingredient Variation Tip: For a citrusy twist, add a drizzle of balsamic vinegar or lemon juice before serving. This will introduce a tangy flavor that complements the sweetness of the oranges and the crispness of the fennel beautifully.

Green Bean Almondine

Preparation Time: 10 minutes
Cooking Time: 10 minutes
Ingredients:
- 1 lb fresh green beans, trimmed
- 2 tablespoons sliced almonds
- 2 tablespoons unsalted butter
- Salt and pepper to taste
- Lemon zest (for garnish, optional)
Instructions:
1. Bring a large pot of salted water to a boil. Add the green beans and cook until they are tender but still crisp, about 5 minutes. Drain and immediately plunge the beans into ice water to stop the cooking process. Drain again and set aside.
2. In a dry skillet over medium heat, toast the sliced almonds, stirring frequently, until they are golden brown and fragrant, about 3 minutes. Remove from the skillet and set aside.
3. In the same skillet, melt the butter over medium heat. Add the blanched green beans, salt, and pepper. Cook, stirring occasionally, until the beans are heated through, about 5 minutes.
4. Transfer the green beans to a serving dish. Sprinkle with the toasted almonds and lemon zest if using. Serve immediately.
Macronutrients:
- **kcal:** 160
- **Carbs:** 10g
- **Protein:** 4g
- **Fat:** 12g
- **Potassium:** 239mg
- **Calcium:** 55mg
- **Magnesium:** 30mg
Ingredient Variation Tip: For a vegan version, substitute the butter with olive oil. To add a savory twist, include a clove of minced garlic when sautéing the green beans in butter or oil.

Lemon Dill Cucumber Salad

Preparation time: 10 minutes

Cooking time: 0 minutes

Ingredients:
- 2 large cucumbers, thinly sliced
- 1/4 cup fresh dill, chopped
- 2 tablespoons olive oil
- 1 tablespoon lemon juice
- Salt and pepper to taste

Instructions:
1. In a large mixing bowl, combine the thinly sliced cucumbers and chopped fresh dill.
2. In a small bowl, whisk together the olive oil and lemon juice until well combined. Season with salt and pepper to taste.
3. Pour the olive oil and lemon juice dressing over the cucumber and dill mixture. Toss gently to ensure all the slices are evenly coated.
4. Serve immediately, or chill in the refrigerator for about 15 minutes before serving for a refreshing touch.

Macronutrients:
- **Kcal:** 120
- **Carbs:** 6g
- **Protein:** 1g
- **Fat:** 10g
- **Potassium:** 230mg
- **Calcium:** 30mg
- **Magnesium:** 22mg

Ingredient Variation Tip: For an added crunch and nutritional boost, sprinkle some chopped walnuts or almonds over the salad before serving.

Peach and Arugula Salad

Preparation time: 5 minutes

Cooking time: 0 minutes

Ingredients:
- 2 cups arugula
- 1 large peach, sliced
- 1/4 cup crumbled feta cheese
- 2 tablespoons balsamic glaze
- 1 tablespoon olive oil

Instructions:
1. In a large salad bowl, combine the arugula and sliced peach.
2. Drizzle the olive oil over the salad and gently toss to coat the arugula and peach slices evenly.
3. Sprinkle the crumbled feta cheese over the salad.
4. Drizzle the balsamic glaze over the top of the salad just before serving.

Macronutrients:
- **Kcal:** 180
- **Carbs:** 15g
- **Protein:** 4g
- **Fat:** 12g
- **Potassium:** 200mg
- **Calcium:** 150mg
- **Magnesium:** 30mg

Ingredient Variation Tip: For a crunchy addition, sprinkle toasted walnuts or almonds over the salad before serving. This not only adds texture but also complements the sweetness of the peach and the tanginess of the feta cheese.

Radish and Cucumber Salad

Preparation time: 10 minutes

Cooking time: 0 minutes

Ingredients:
- 1 cup radishes, thinly sliced
- 1 large cucumber, thinly sliced
- 2 tablespoons olive oil
- 1 tablespoon white wine vinegar
- Salt and pepper to taste

Instructions:
1. In a large mixing bowl, combine the thinly sliced radishes and cucumber.
2. Drizzle the olive oil and white wine vinegar over the sliced vegetables. Gently toss to ensure all slices are evenly coated.
3. Season with salt and pepper to taste. Toss again to distribute the seasoning evenly.
4. Chill in the refrigerator for about 5 minutes before serving to allow the flavors to meld together.

Macronutrients:
- **kcal:** 120
- **Carbs:** 6g
- **Protein:** 1g
- **Fat:** 10g
- **Potassium:** 270mg
- **Calcium:** 30mg
- **Magnesium:** 24mg

Ingredient Variation Tip: For an added crunch and a pop of color, sprinkle some chopped walnuts or almonds over the salad before serving.

Watermelon Feta Salad

Preparation time: 5 minutes

Cooking time: 0 minutes

Ingredients:
- 4 cups cubed watermelon
- 1/2 cup crumbled feta cheese
- 1/4 cup fresh mint leaves, chopped
- 2 tablespoons balsamic glaze
- Salt to taste

Instructions:
1. In a large bowl, combine the cubed watermelon and crumbled feta cheese.
2. Gently toss the watermelon and feta with the chopped fresh mint leaves. Season with a pinch of salt to enhance the flavors.
3. Drizzle the balsamic glaze over the salad just before serving, ensuring an even distribution for a touch of sweetness and acidity.
4. Serve the salad immediately, or chill in the refrigerator for about 15 minutes for a refreshing summer dish.

Macronutrients:
- **kcal:** 120
- **Carbs:** 18g
- **Protein:** 4g
- **Fat:** 4.5g
- **Potassium:** 170mg
- **Calcium:** 100mg
- **Magnesium:** 15mg

Ingredient Variation Tip: For a crunchy texture, add a handful of toasted pine nuts or walnuts to the salad before serving. This not only introduces a new flavor dimension but also adds healthy fats and nutrients.

Desserts Recipes

Almond Butter Cookies

Preparation Time: 10 minutes
Cooking Time: 12 minutes
Ingredients:
- 1 cup almond butter
- 3/4 cup sugar
- 1 large egg
- 1 teaspoon baking soda
- 1/2 teaspoon vanilla extract

Instructions:
1. Preheat the oven to 350°F (175°C). Line a baking sheet with parchment paper.
2. In a mixing bowl, combine almond butter, sugar, egg, baking soda, and vanilla extract. Stir until the mixture is smooth and well combined.
3. Scoop tablespoon-sized balls of dough onto the prepared baking sheet, spacing them about 2 inches apart.
4. Bake in the preheated oven for 10-12 minutes, or until the cookies are golden around the edges. Allow them to cool on the baking sheet for 5 minutes before transferring to a wire rack to cool completely.

Macronutrients:
- **Kcal:** 160
- **Carbs:** 14g
- **Protein:** 4g
- **Fat:** 10g
- **Potassium:** 120mg
- **Calcium:** 60mg
- **Magnesium:** 75mg

Ingredient Variation Tip: For a chocolatey twist, mix in 1/2 cup of dark chocolate chips into the dough before baking. This adds a rich flavor and texture contrast to the soft and chewy almond butter cookies.

Apple Cinnamon Bites

Preparation Time: 10 minutes
Cooking Time: 15 minutes
Ingredients:
- 2 large apples, peeled, cored, and diced
- 1 tablespoon ground cinnamon
- 2 tablespoons honey
- 1/4 cup water
- 1 tablespoon unsalted butter

Instructions:
1. In a medium saucepan, combine the diced apples, ground cinnamon, honey, and water. Stir well to ensure the apples are evenly coated with cinnamon and honey.
2. Place the saucepan over medium heat and bring the mixture to a simmer. Cover and cook for about 10 minutes, stirring occasionally, until the apples are soft.
3. Uncover the saucepan and stir in the unsalted butter until it's completely melted and mixed into the apple mixture. Cook for an additional 5 minutes, or until the mixture thickens slightly.
4. Remove from heat and allow the apple cinnamon bites to cool slightly before serving.

Macronutrients:
- **Kcal:** 150
- **Carbs:** 34g
- **Protein:** 0.5g
- **Fat:** 2g
- **Potassium:** 194mg
- **Calcium:** 20mg
- **Magnesium:** 8mg

Ingredient Variation Tip: For a nutty flavor and extra crunch, add a handful of chopped walnuts or pecans to the mixture during the last 5 minutes of cooking.

Berry Chia Pudding

Preparation Time: 5 minutes
Cooking Time: 0 minutes
Ingredients:
- 1 cup unsweetened almond milk
- 1/2 cup chia seeds
- 1 tablespoon honey (or maple syrup for a vegan option)
- 1/2 teaspoon vanilla extract
- 1 cup mixed berries (fresh or frozen)

Instructions:
1. In a mixing bowl, whisk together the almond milk, chia seeds, honey (or maple syrup), and vanilla extract until well combined.
2. Pour the mixture into a jar or container and refrigerate for at least 4 hours, or overnight, until it has thickened and the chia seeds have absorbed the liquid, creating a pudding-like consistency.
3. Before serving, stir the pudding to ensure it's evenly mixed. If the pudding is too thick, you can add a little more almond milk to reach your desired consistency.
4. Top the chia pudding with mixed berries. Serve chilled.

Macronutrients:
- **Kcal:** 295
- **Carbs:** 34g
- **Protein:** 8g
- **Fat:** 15g
- **Potassium:** 200mg
- **Calcium:** 350mg
- **Magnesium:** 95mg

Ingredient Variation Tip: For an added nutritional boost, sprinkle a tablespoon of flaxseeds or hemp seeds on top of the pudding before serving. This not only enhances the fiber content but also adds healthy omega-3 fatty acids.

Chocolate Avocado Mousse

Preparation Time: 5 minutes
Cooking Time: 0 minutes
Ingredients:
- 2 ripe avocados, peeled and pitted
- 1/4 cup cocoa powder
- 1/4 cup honey or maple syrup (for vegan option)
- 1/2 teaspoon vanilla extract
- Pinch of salt

Instructions:
1. Place the peeled and pitted avocados in a blender or food processor. Add the cocoa powder, honey (or maple syrup for a vegan version), vanilla extract, and a pinch of salt.
2. Blend on high until the mixture is completely smooth. Pause to scrape down the sides of the blender or food processor as needed to ensure all ingredients are well incorporated.
3. Taste the mousse and adjust sweetness if necessary by adding a little more honey or maple syrup. Blend again if additional sweetener is added.
4. Transfer the mousse to serving dishes and refrigerate for at least 1 hour to chill and set before serving.

Macronutrients:
- **Kcal:** 320
- **Carbs:** 35g
- **Protein:** 4g
- **Fat:** 20g
- **Potassium:** 487mg
- **Calcium:** 20mg
- **Magnesium:** 45mg

Ingredient Variation Tip: For an extra flavor boost, mix in a pinch of cinnamon or chili powder before blending. This will add a subtle warmth and depth to the chocolate mousse.

Coconut Macaroons

Preparation Time: 10 minutes
Cooking Time: 15 minutes
Ingredients:
- 2 large egg whites
- 1/4 cup honey
- 1/2 teaspoon vanilla extract
- 2 cups unsweetened shredded coconut
- Pinch of salt

Instructions:
1. Preheat your oven to 325°F (163°C) and line a baking sheet with parchment paper.
2. In a mixing bowl, whisk together the egg whites, honey, vanilla extract, and a pinch of salt until well combined. Stir in the shredded coconut until the mixture is evenly moistened.
3. Using a spoon or a cookie scoop, form the mixture into small mounds on the prepared baking sheet, spacing them about an inch apart.
4. Bake in the preheated oven for 15 minutes, or until the macaroons are golden around the edges. Let them cool on the baking sheet for 5 minutes before transferring to a wire rack to cool completely.

Macronutrients:
- **Kcal:** 130
- **Carbs:** 10g
- **Protein:** 2g
- **Fat:** 9g
- **Potassium:** 90mg
- **Calcium:** 10mg
- **Magnesium:** 20mg

Ingredient Variation Tip: For a chocolate-dipped version, melt dark chocolate and dip the bottom of each cooled macaroon into the chocolate, then place on parchment paper until the chocolate sets.

Greek Yogurt Bark

Preparation Time: 5 minutes

Cooking Time: 2 hours (freezing time)

Ingredients:
- 2 cups plain Greek yogurt
- 3 tablespoons honey
- 1/2 cup mixed berries (such as strawberries, blueberries, and raspberries), fresh or frozen
- 1/4 cup sliced almonds
- 1 tablespoon dark chocolate chips

Instructions:
1. In a medium bowl, mix the Greek yogurt with honey until well combined. Spread the mixture evenly onto a baking sheet lined with parchment paper, creating a thickness of about 1/2 inch.
2. Sprinkle the mixed berries, sliced almonds, and dark chocolate chips over the yogurt layer.
3. Place the baking sheet in the freezer and freeze for at least 2 hours, or until the yogurt bark is fully frozen and solid.
4. Break the frozen yogurt bark into pieces. Serve immediately or store in an airtight container in the freezer for up to 1 month.

Macronutrients:
- **Kcal:** 180
- **Carbs:** 22g
- **Protein:** 10g
- **Fat:** 7g
- **Potassium:** 240mg
- **Calcium:** 120mg
- **Magnesium:** 30mg

Ingredient Variation Tip: For a tropical twist, substitute mixed berries with diced mango, pineapple, and shredded coconut.

Lemon Ricotta Cheesecake

Preparation Time: 10 minutes

Cooking Time: 0 minutes

Ingredients:
- 1 cup ricotta cheese
- 1/4 cup honey
- Zest of 1 lemon
- 1 teaspoon vanilla extract
- 4 graham crackers, crushed

Instructions:
1. In a medium bowl, mix together the ricotta cheese, honey, lemon zest, and vanilla extract until well combined and smooth.
2. Spoon the ricotta mixture into serving dishes, creating an even layer at the bottom.
3. Refrigerate for at least 10 minutes to allow the flavors to meld together and the mixture to chill.
4. Just before serving, sprinkle the crushed graham crackers over the top of each cheesecake serving for a crunchy texture.

Macronutrients:
- **Kcal:** 220
- **Carbs:** 28g
- **Protein:** 10g
- **Fat:** 8g
- **Potassium:** 42mg
- **Calcium:** 159mg
- **Magnesium:** 8mg

Ingredient Variation Tip: For a nuttier flavor and extra crunch, mix in or top with chopped almonds or walnuts instead of graham crackers.

Peach Yogurt Pops

Preparation Time: 5 minutes

Cooking Time: 0 minutes (Freeze time: 4 hours)

Ingredients:
- 2 cups Greek yogurt (plain, non-fat)
- 1 cup fresh peaches, diced
- 2 tablespoons honey
- 1 teaspoon vanilla extract
- Popsicle sticks

Instructions:
1. In a blender, combine Greek yogurt, fresh peaches, honey, and vanilla extract. Blend until the mixture is smooth.
2. Pour the mixture into popsicle molds, leaving a little space at the top for expansion. Insert popsicle sticks into the center of each mold.
3. Freeze the popsicles for at least 4 hours, or until they are completely solid.
4. To release the popsicles from the molds, run warm water over the outside of the molds for a few seconds, then gently pull the sticks.

Macronutrients:
- **Kcal:** 120
- **Carbs:** 18g
- **Protein:** 8g
- **Fat:** 0g
- **Potassium:** 200mg
- **Calcium:** 100mg
- **Magnesium:** 20mg

Ingredient Variation Tip: For a tropical twist, substitute peaches with mango or pineapple. This will give the yogurt pops a vibrant, exotic flavor that's perfect for summer.

Strawberry Banana Smoothie Bowl

Preparation Time: 5 minutes

Cooking Time: 0 minutes

Ingredients:
- 1 cup frozen strawberries
- 1 ripe banana
- 1/2 cup Greek yogurt (plain, non-fat)
- 1/4 cup almond milk
- Toppings: Sliced strawberries, banana slices, and a sprinkle of granola

Instructions:
1. In a blender, combine the frozen strawberries, ripe banana, Greek yogurt, and almond milk. Blend on high until smooth and creamy.
2. Pour the smoothie mixture into a bowl.
3. Arrange the sliced strawberries, banana slices, and a sprinkle of granola on top of the smoothie bowl.
4. Serve immediately for a refreshing and nutritious breakfast or snack.

Macronutrients:
- **Kcal:** 280
- **Carbs:** 52g
- **Protein:** 15g
- **Fat:** 3g
- **Potassium:** 750mg
- **Calcium:** 150mg
- **Magnesium:** 60mg

Ingredient Variation Tip: For a vegan version, substitute Greek yogurt with a plant-based yogurt alternative. To add extra protein, sprinkle chia seeds or hemp seeds on top of the smoothie bowl.

Vanilla Panna Cotta

Preparation Time: 10 minutes

Cooking Time: 10 minutes

Ingredients:
- 2 cups heavy cream
- 1/4 cup sugar
- 1 teaspoon vanilla extract
- 2 teaspoons gelatin powder
- 3 tablespoons cold water

Instructions:
1. In a small bowl, sprinkle the gelatin over the cold water and let it sit for about 5 minutes to soften.
2. In a saucepan, combine the heavy cream and sugar. Cook over medium heat, stirring until the sugar is completely dissolved. Do not let it boil.
3. Remove the cream mixture from the heat and add the softened gelatin. Stir until the gelatin is completely dissolved. Mix in the vanilla extract.
4. Pour the mixture into 4 serving glasses or ramekins. Chill in the refrigerator for at least 4 hours, or until set.

Macronutrients:
- **Kcal:** 410
- **Carbs:** 16g
- **Protein:** 3g
- **Fat:** 36g
- **Potassium:** 99mg
- **Calcium:** 78mg
- **Magnesium:** 12mg

Ingredient Variation Tip: For a citrus twist, add the zest of 1 lemon or orange to the cream mixture before chilling. This will infuse the panna cotta with a refreshing citrus flavor.

Chapter 5: Lifestyle Tips for Heart Health

Embarking on a journey to better heart health involves more than just mindful eating; it requires embracing a holistic lifestyle that nurtures your entire well-being. This chapter delves into essential lifestyle habits that, when combined with the Mediterranean DASH diet, can significantly enhance your cardiovascular health. We'll explore the importance of regular physical activity, effective stress management techniques, and the role of quality sleep in maintaining a healthy heart. Additionally, we'll discuss the benefits of staying hydrated and the impact of smoking and alcohol on heart health. These practical tips are designed to seamlessly integrate into your daily routine, making it easier to sustain long-term healthy habits. By adopting these lifestyle changes, you'll not only support your heart but also improve your overall quality of life, paving the way for a happier, healthier you.

Incorporating Physical Activity

A heart-healthy lifestyle is built on the foundation of both nutritious eating and regular physical activity. Combining the Mediterranean DASH diet with consistent exercise amplifies the benefits of each, leading to improved cardiovascular health, better weight management, and enhanced overall well-being. This section will guide you through understanding the importance of physical activity, how to integrate it into your daily routine, and tips for staying motivated and safe.

The Importance of Physical Activity for Heart Health

Regular physical activity offers numerous benefits for the heart:

- **Strengthens the Heart Muscle:** Like any muscle, the heart becomes stronger and more efficient with exercise, improving its ability to pump blood throughout the body.

- **Improves Blood Pressure:** Exercise helps lower high blood pressure, a significant risk factor for heart disease.

- **Enhances Cholesterol Levels:** Physical activity can increase high-density lipoprotein (HDL) cholesterol (the "good" cholesterol) and decrease low-density lipoprotein (LDL) cholesterol (the "bad" cholesterol).

- **Aids in Weight Management:** Burning calories through exercise helps maintain a healthy weight, reducing strain on the heart.

- **Reduces Stress:** Physical activity releases endorphins, natural mood lifters that can reduce stress and anxiety levels.

Types of Heart-Healthy Exercises

Incorporate a mix of the following exercise types for a balanced fitness routine:

1. Aerobic (Cardio) Exercises

These activities increase your heart rate and breathing, improving cardiovascular endurance.

- **Examples:** Walking, jogging, swimming, cycling, dancing, and aerobic classes.
- **Recommendations:** Aim for at least 150 minutes of moderate-intensity or 75 minutes of vigorous-intensity aerobic exercise per week, as per health guidelines.

2. Strength Training

Building muscle mass boosts metabolism and supports joint health.

- **Examples:** Weightlifting, resistance band exercises, bodyweight workouts like push-ups and squats.
- **Recommendations:** Include strength training exercises at least two days per week, targeting all major muscle groups.

3. Flexibility and Balance Exercises

These activities enhance the range of motion and prevent injuries.

- **Examples:** Stretching routines, yoga, tai chi, and Pilates.
- **Recommendations:** Incorporate flexibility and balance exercises into your routine several times a week.

Integrating Physical Activity into Your Daily Routine

Finding time for exercise can be challenging, but with some creativity, you can make it a natural part of your day:

- **Start Small:** Begin with short sessions, like 10-minute walks, and gradually increase duration and intensity.
- **Active Commuting:** Walk or cycle to work or while running errands whenever possible.
- **Take the Stairs:** Opt for stairs over elevators to add more activity to your day.
- **Scheduled Workouts:** Block out specific times in your calendar for exercise, treating it like any other important appointment.
- **Social Activities:** Join a sports team, walking group, or exercise class to make physical activity more enjoyable and accountable.
- **Incorporate Activity at Home:** Engage in active household chores like gardening, vacuuming, or washing the car.

Staying Motivated

Maintaining motivation is key to making exercise a lifelong habit:

- **Set Realistic Goals:** Define clear, achievable objectives, such as walking 30 minutes a day, five days a week.

- **Track Progress:** Use a journal or fitness app to record your activities and celebrate milestones.

- **Find Enjoyable Activities:** Choose exercises you enjoy to increase the likelihood of sticking with them.

- **Workout Buddy:** Partner with a friend or family member to stay accountable and make exercising more fun.

- **Variety is Key:** Mix up your routine to prevent boredom and work different muscle groups.

Safety Tips

Prioritize safety to make your exercise routine effective and injury-free:

- **Consult a Professional:** Before starting any new exercise program, especially if you have existing health conditions, consult with a healthcare provider.

- **Warm-Up and Cool-Down:** Begin with light activity to prepare your body and end with stretching to aid recovery.

- **Listen to Your Body:** Pay attention to signs of overexertion, such as dizziness or shortness of breath, and adjust accordingly.

- **Stay Hydrated:** Drink plenty of water before, during, and after exercise.

- **Proper Equipment:** Use appropriate footwear and gear to support your activities and prevent injuries.

Combining Diet and Exercise for Optimal Heart Health

Pairing your physical activity routine with the Mediterranean DASH diet creates a powerful synergy:

- **Enhanced Weight Loss:** Balanced nutrition fuels your workouts, while exercise helps regulate appetite and boosts metabolism.

- **Improved Nutrient Utilization:** Physical activity can enhance the body's ability to utilize the nutrients from your heart-healthy diet.

- **Better Blood Pressure Control:** Diet and exercise work together to reduce hypertension more effectively than either alone.

Sample Weekly Exercise Plan

Here's a simple plan to help you get started:

- **Monday:** 30-minute brisk walk (aerobic)

- **Tuesday:** Strength training session focusing on upper body

- **Wednesday:** Yoga class (flexibility and balance)

- **Thursday:** 30-minute cycling or swimming (aerobic)
- **Friday:** Strength training session focusing on lower body
- **Saturday:** Group sport or hike (aerobic and social activity)
- **Sunday:** Rest day with light stretching or a leisurely walk

Stress Management Techniques

Managing stress is a crucial component of maintaining heart health. Chronic stress can have detrimental effects on the cardiovascular system, contributing to high blood pressure, heart disease, and other health issues. This section explores the relationship between stress and heart health, helps you recognize stress signals, and provides practical techniques to manage stress effectively. By incorporating these strategies into your daily routine, you can enhance your overall well-being and support your journey toward a healthier heart.

The Impact of Stress on Heart Health

Stress triggers a series of physiological responses known as the "fight or flight" reaction, releasing hormones like adrenaline and cortisol. While these responses are helpful in short-term situations, chronic stress keeps the body in a heightened state, leading to:

- **Increased Blood Pressure:** Stress hormones cause blood vessels to constrict, raising blood pressure and forcing the heart to work harder.
- **Elevated Heart Rate:** Prolonged elevated heart rate can strain the heart and lead to arrhythmias.
- **Inflammation:** Chronic stress can contribute to inflammation in the arteries, promoting the buildup of plaque.
- **Unhealthy Behaviors:** Stress often leads to coping mechanisms like overeating, smoking, or excessive alcohol consumption, which further harm heart health.

Recognizing Stress and Its Symptoms

Identifying stress is the first step toward managing it. Common signs of stress include:

- **Emotional Symptoms:** Anxiety, irritability, depression, restlessness.
- **Physical Symptoms:** Headaches, muscle tension, fatigue, sleep disturbances.
- **Cognitive Symptoms:** Difficulty concentrating, racing thoughts, forgetfulness.
- **Behavioral Symptoms:** Changes in appetite, withdrawal from social activities, procrastination.

Effective Stress Management Techniques

Implementing stress-reduction strategies can mitigate the harmful effects of stress on your heart. Here are some evidence-based techniques:

1. Mindfulness and Meditation

Mindfulness involves being fully present in the moment, acknowledging thoughts and feelings without judgment.

- **Benefits:** Reduces stress hormones, lowers blood pressure, improves emotional regulation.
- **How to Practice:**
    - **Mindful Breathing:** Focus on your breath, noticing each inhale and exhale.
    - **Body Scan Meditation:** Progressively focus on different parts of your body, releasing tension.
    - **Mindful Observation:** Engage your senses by paying close attention to sights, sounds, or sensations around you.

2. Deep Breathing Exercises

Deep breathing activates the body's relaxation response.

- **Benefits:** Lowers heart rate and blood pressure, reduces anxiety.
- **How to Practice:**
    - **Diaphragmatic Breathing:** Breathe in slowly through your nose, allowing your abdomen to expand, then exhale slowly through your mouth.
    - **4-7-8 Technique:** Inhale for 4 seconds, hold for 7 seconds, exhale for 8 seconds.

3. Physical Activity for Stress Relief

Exercise not only benefits the heart physically but also reduces stress.

- **Benefits:** Releases endorphins, improves mood, enhances sleep quality.
- **How to Practice:**
    - Engage in activities you enjoy, such as walking, yoga, swimming, or dancing.
    - Even short bursts of activity, like a 10-minute walk, can alleviate stress.

4. Time Management and Prioritization

Effective time management reduces feelings of overwhelm.

- **Benefits:** Increases productivity, reduces anxiety about deadlines and obligations.
- **How to Practice:**

- o **Create a Schedule:** Use planners or digital calendars to organize tasks.
- o **Set Priorities:** Focus on important tasks and delegate when possible.
- o **Break Tasks into Smaller Steps:** Tackling tasks piece by piece makes them more manageable.

5. Social Support and Communication

Connecting with others provides emotional support.

- **Benefits:** Reduces feelings of isolation, offers new perspectives on problems.
- **How to Practice:**
  - o **Reach Out:** Talk to friends or family members about your feelings.
  - o **Join Groups:** Participate in community activities or support groups.
  - o **Quality Time:** Schedule regular interactions with loved ones.

6. Relaxation Techniques

Practicing relaxation helps counteract stress responses.

- **Benefits:** Lowers muscle tension, decreases stress hormones.
- **How to Practice:**
  - o **Progressive Muscle Relaxation:** Tense and then relax different muscle groups sequentially.
  - o **Guided Imagery:** Visualize calming scenes or experiences.
  - o **Aromatherapy:** Use essential oils like lavender or chamomile to promote relaxation.

7. Hobbies and Leisure Activities

Engaging in enjoyable activities distracts from stressors.

- **Benefits:** Enhances mood, provides a sense of accomplishment.
- **How to Practice:**
  - o **Creative Pursuits:** Painting, writing, playing music.
  - o **Outdoor Activities:** Gardening, hiking, bird-watching.
  - o **Mind-engaging Games:** Puzzles, chess, or other strategy games.

8. Professional Help When Needed

Recognizing when to seek help is a sign of strength.

- **Benefits:** Provides personalized strategies, addresses underlying issues.

- **How to Practice:**
    - **Therapy:** Consult a psychologist or counselor for cognitive-behavioral therapy or other modalities.
    - **Stress Management Programs:** Enroll in workshops or courses.
    - **Medical Consultation:** Discuss stress symptoms with your healthcare provider.

Incorporating Stress Management into Daily Life

Making stress reduction a part of your routine enhances its effectiveness.

- **Morning Rituals:** Start your day with meditation or gentle stretching.
- **Mindful Moments:** Take short breaks during the day to practice deep breathing.
- **Evening Wind-Down:** Establish a relaxing bedtime routine, such as reading or taking a warm bath.
- **Digital Detox:** Limit screen time, especially before bed, to reduce overstimulation.
- **Set Boundaries:** Learn to say no to additional commitments that overload your schedule.

Combining Stress Management with Diet and Exercise

An integrated approach maximizes heart health benefits.

- **Synergy with Diet:** Certain foods can help reduce stress levels. Incorporate stress-relieving foods like:
    - **Omega-3 Fatty Acids:** Found in salmon, walnuts, flaxseeds.
    - **Antioxidant-Rich Foods:** Berries, dark chocolate, leafy greens.
    - **Herbal Teas:** Chamomile, green tea, which have calming properties.
- **Enhancing Exercise Benefits:** Mind-body exercises like yoga and tai chi combine physical activity with mindfulness.

Tips for Sustained Stress Management

- **Regular Practice:** Consistency is key. Schedule stress management activities like any other important task.
- **Personalization:** Choose techniques that resonate with you for greater effectiveness.
- **Progress Tracking:** Keep a journal to note stress levels and what strategies work best.
- **Patience:** Developing new habits takes time. Be patient with yourself as you incorporate these techniques.

Importance of Hydration and Sleep

Achieving optimal heart health extends beyond diet and exercise; it also involves maintaining proper hydration and ensuring adequate sleep. Both hydration and sleep play crucial roles in cardiovascular function, overall wellness, and the body's ability to recover and regenerate. This chapter explores the significant impact that hydration and sleep have on heart health, provides practical tips for staying hydrated, and offers strategies for improving sleep quality. By understanding and prioritizing these often-overlooked aspects of health, you can further support your journey toward a healthier heart.

The Role of Hydration in Heart Health

Proper hydration is essential for the efficient functioning of every system in the body, including the cardiovascular system. Water makes up about 60% of the human body and is vital for various physiological processes.

How Hydration Affects the Heart

- **Blood Volume Regulation:** Adequate hydration maintains the proper volume of blood, which is crucial for optimal blood pressure and circulation.

- **Heart Function Efficiency:** Dehydration can cause the heart to work harder to pump blood, leading to increased heart rate and potential strain.

- **Electrolyte Balance:** Fluids help maintain the balance of minerals like sodium and potassium, essential for normal heart rhythm and muscle contractions.

- **Temperature Regulation:** Water aids in regulating body temperature, preventing overheating during physical activity, which can stress the heart.

Consequences of Dehydration

- **Increased Blood Viscosity:** Dehydration thickens the blood, making it more difficult for the heart to circulate it efficiently.

- **Elevated Heart Rate and Blood Pressure:** The heart compensates for lower blood volume by beating faster, potentially raising blood pressure.

- **Impaired Cognitive Function:** Dehydration can affect concentration and mood, indirectly influencing stress levels and heart health.

Tips for Staying Hydrated

Ensuring adequate fluid intake is a simple yet effective way to support heart health.

Daily Hydration Guidelines

- **General Recommendations:** While individual needs vary, a common guideline is about 8 cups (64 ounces) of water per day for adults. However, factors like age, gender, activity level, and climate can affect requirements.

- **Listen to Your Body:** Thirst is a natural indicator, but don't rely solely on it; by the time you feel thirsty, you might already be mildly dehydrated.
- **Monitor Urine Color:** Pale yellow urine typically indicates proper hydration, while darker urine suggests the need for more fluids.

Hydration Strategies

- **Start Early:** Drink a glass of water first thing in the morning to replenish fluids lost overnight.
- **Carry a Water Bottle:** Keeping water accessible encourages regular sipping throughout the day.
- **Set Reminders:** Use alarms or apps to prompt you to drink water at regular intervals.
- **Flavor Your Water:** Add slices of citrus fruits, cucumbers, or herbs like mint to enhance the taste naturally.
- **Include Hydrating Foods:** Consume fruits and vegetables with high water content, such as watermelon, cucumbers, oranges, and strawberries.
- **Limit Diuretics:** Be mindful of beverages like coffee and alcohol that can increase fluid loss.

Hydration During Exercise

- **Pre-Exercise:** Drink water about 2 hours before physical activity.
- **During Exercise:** Sip water every 15–20 minutes, especially during prolonged or intense workouts.
- **Post-Exercise:** Rehydrate after activity to replace fluids lost through sweat.

The Impact of Sleep on Heart Health

Quality sleep is as vital to health as proper nutrition and exercise. Sleep allows the body to repair itself, supports brain function, and plays a significant role in maintaining heart health.

How Sleep Affects the Heart

- **Blood Pressure Regulation:** During sleep, blood pressure naturally dips. Insufficient sleep can prevent this nightly drop, leading to hypertension.
- **Heart Rate Variability:** Sleep impacts heart rate variability, an indicator of cardiovascular fitness and resilience.
- **Hormonal Balance:** Sleep influences the production of hormones related to stress, appetite, and glucose metabolism, all affecting heart health.
- **Inflammation Reduction:** Adequate sleep helps reduce inflammatory markers associated with heart disease.

Consequences of Poor Sleep

- **Increased Risk of Heart Disease:** Chronic sleep deprivation is linked to higher incidences of hypertension, coronary heart disease, and stroke.

- **Weight Gain:** Lack of sleep can disrupt hormones that regulate hunger, leading to overeating and weight gain, further stressing the heart.

- **Impaired Glucose Metabolism:** Poor sleep affects insulin sensitivity, increasing the risk of type 2 diabetes, a risk factor for heart disease.

Tips for Improving Sleep Quality

Prioritizing sleep hygiene can enhance sleep quality and duration, positively impacting heart health.

Establish a Consistent Sleep Schedule

- **Regular Bedtime and Wake Time:** Go to bed and wake up at the same times every day, even on weekends, to regulate your body's internal clock.

- **Sleep Duration:** Aim for 7–9 hours of sleep per night, as recommended for most adults.

Create a Sleep-Conducive Environment

- **Comfortable Bedding:** Invest in a supportive mattress and comfortable pillows.

- **Optimal Room Temperature:** Keep the bedroom cool, around 65°F (18°C), to promote restful sleep.

- **Dark and Quiet:** Use blackout curtains or a sleep mask to block light, and earplugs or white noise machines to reduce noise disturbances.

- **Electronic Device-Free Zone:** Remove TVs, computers, and smartphones from the bedroom to minimize distractions and blue light exposure.

Establish a Relaxing Pre-Sleep Routine

- **Wind-Down Activities:** Engage in calming activities before bed, such as reading, gentle stretching, or taking a warm bath.

- **Avoid Stimulants:** Limit caffeine and nicotine intake, especially in the afternoon and evening.

- **Limit Alcohol:** While alcohol may induce sleepiness, it can disrupt sleep patterns and reduce sleep quality.

Mind Your Diet

- **Evening Meals:** Avoid heavy or spicy meals close to bedtime, which can cause discomfort and disrupt sleep.

- **Hydration Balance:** While staying hydrated is important, reduce fluid intake before bed to minimize nighttime awakenings for bathroom visits.

Manage Stress

- **Relaxation Techniques:** Practice deep breathing, meditation, or progressive muscle relaxation to ease into sleep.

- **Journaling:** Write down worries or a to-do list to clear your mind before bed.

Physical Activity

- **Regular Exercise:** Engage in physical activity during the day to promote better sleep but avoid vigorous workouts close to bedtime.

- **Morning Sunlight Exposure:** Natural light helps regulate circadian rhythms, improving sleep patterns.

Seek Professional Help if Needed

- **Sleep Disorders:** If you suspect a sleep disorder like sleep apnea or insomnia, consult a healthcare professional for evaluation and treatment.

Hydration and Sleep: A Balancing Act

Hydration and sleep are interconnected, and balancing both is essential.

Nighttime Hydration Tips

- **Stay Hydrated During the Day:** Focus on fluid intake throughout the day to avoid excessive thirst at night.

- **Evening Fluid Intake:** Reduce water consumption 1–2 hours before bed to prevent nocturnal awakenings.

Addressing Nocturia

- **Nocturia (Frequent Nighttime Urination):** Can disrupt sleep and affect heart health indirectly.

- **Strategies:**
    - Limit evening beverages.
    - Empty your bladder before bed.
    - Discuss with a doctor if nocturia persists, as it may indicate underlying health issues.

Integrating Hydration and Sleep with the Mediterranean DASH Diet

Combining proper hydration and quality sleep with the Mediterranean DASH diet enhances heart health benefits.

Dietary Considerations

- **Hydrating Foods:** The diet includes plenty of fruits and vegetables that contribute to hydration.

- **Sleep-Promoting Nutrients:**

  - **Magnesium:** Found in leafy greens, nuts, and whole grains, supports sleep quality.

  - **Tryptophan:** An amino acid in turkey, fish, and dairy, can promote sleepiness.

  - **Complex Carbohydrates:** Whole grains can increase serotonin levels, aiding sleep.

Alcohol and Caffeine Intake

- **Moderation is Key:** The Mediterranean diet allows moderate alcohol consumption, typically red wine. Excessive intake can disrupt sleep and hydration.

- **Caffeine Awareness:** Limit coffee and tea intake in the late afternoon and evening.

Monitoring and Adjusting

Stay attentive to how your body responds to hydration and sleep patterns.

- **Keep a Journal:** Track fluid intake, sleep duration, and quality to identify patterns and make adjustments.

- **Listen to Your Body:** Pay attention to signals of dehydration or sleep deprivation and respond accordingly.

Monitoring Blood Pressure at Home

Monitoring your blood pressure at home is a valuable practice for managing hypertension and maintaining heart health. Regular home measurements provide insights into how your daily activities, diet, and stress levels affect your blood pressure. This chapter guides you through the importance of home monitoring, how to choose the right equipment, proper measurement techniques, and how to interpret and track your readings. By becoming proactive in monitoring, you empower yourself to make informed decisions and collaborate effectively with your healthcare provider.

Why Monitor Blood Pressure at Home?

Benefits of Home Monitoring

- **Early Detection:** Identifies hypertension or worsening blood pressure early, allowing for timely intervention.

- **Informed Decisions:** Provides data to adjust lifestyle habits, such as diet and exercise, based on trends.

- **Medication Effectiveness:** Helps assess how well blood pressure medications are working.

- **Eliminates White-Coat Syndrome:** Reduces the effect of anxiety-induced elevated readings that can occur in clinical settings.

- **Empowerment:** Increases awareness and encourages active participation in managing heart health.

Understanding Blood Pressure Readings

- **Systolic Pressure (Top Number):** Measures the pressure in your arteries when the heart beats.

- **Diastolic Pressure (Bottom Number):** Measures the pressure in your arteries between beats.

- **Normal Range:** Generally considered to be less than 120/80 mmHg.

- **Hypertension Threshold:** Consistently elevated readings of 130/80 mmHg or higher.

Choosing a Home Blood Pressure Monitor

Types of Monitors

1. **Upper Arm Monitors:** Most accurate and recommended for home use.

2. **Wrist Monitors:** More portable but can be less accurate; proper positioning is crucial.

3. **Finger Monitors:** Least accurate and not generally recommended.

Features to Consider

- **Cuff Size:** Ensure the cuff fits your upper arm circumference for accurate readings.

- **Ease of Use:** Look for devices with clear displays and simple operation.

- **Memory Storage:** Ability to store readings for tracking trends over time.

- **Validation:** Choose monitors validated by recognized organizations (e.g., American Heart Association).

- **Battery Life and Power Options:** Consider whether it uses batteries, AC power, or both.

Recommendations

- **Consult Healthcare Providers:** Seek advice on suitable models based on your specific needs.

- **Read Reviews and Ratings:** Look for devices with positive user feedback and reliability.

Preparing for Accurate Measurements

Before You Measure

- **Rest:** Sit quietly for at least 5 minutes before measuring.

- **Avoid Influencing Factors:** Do not smoke, exercise, or consume caffeine or alcohol 30 minutes prior.

- **Bladder Emptying:** Use the restroom beforehand; a full bladder can affect readings.

- **Consistent Timing:** Measure at the same times each day, such as morning and evening.

Proper Positioning

- **Seating:** Sit upright in a chair with back support.

- **Arm Support:** Rest your arm on a flat surface so that the upper arm is at heart level.

- **Feet Placement:** Keep both feet flat on the floor; avoid crossing legs.

- **Cuff Placement:** Wrap the cuff snugly around the bare upper arm, about one inch above the bend of the elbow.

How to Measure Blood Pressure Correctly

Step-by-Step Guide

1. **Prepare the Monitor:** Ensure the device is functioning properly and reset if necessary.

2. **Apply the Cuff:** Place it directly on the skin, not over clothing.

3. **Relax:** Take deep breaths and remain still and silent during the measurement.

4. **Start the Monitor:** Press the start button and allow the device to measure without movement.

5. **Record the Reading:** Note both systolic and diastolic numbers, along with the date and time.

6. **Repeat if Advised:** Some guidelines suggest taking two or three measurements one minute apart and averaging the results.

Avoiding Common Mistakes

- **Talking or Moving:** Can lead to inaccurate readings.

- **Incorrect Cuff Size or Placement:** Affects the accuracy; follow the manufacturer's instructions.

- **Irregular Heartbeat:** If you have arrhythmias, consult your doctor for proper monitoring techniques.

Tracking and Interpreting Your Readings

Keeping a Blood Pressure Log

- **Consistency:** Record all readings promptly and accurately.
- **Additional Notes:** Include notes on medications, diet, physical activity, stress levels, or symptoms.
- **Use Tools:** Consider apps or digital logs that can organize and graph your data.

Interpreting Trends

- **Look for Patterns:** Identify times of day or activities that influence your blood pressure.
- **Assessing Variability:** Some fluctuation is normal, but significant changes should be noted.
- **Consulting Professionals:** Share your log with your healthcare provider for expert interpretation.

When to Seek Medical Advice

Concerning Readings

- **Hypertensive Crisis:** A reading of 180/120 mmHg or higher requires immediate medical attention.
- **Consistently High Readings:** Regular measurements above 130/80 mmHg warrant a discussion with your doctor.
- **Symptoms of Concern:** Dizziness, blurred vision, shortness of breath, or chest pain alongside abnormal readings.

Regular Check-Ups

- **Routine Appointments:** Maintain scheduled visits even if readings are normal.
- **Medication Adjustments:** Use your data to inform potential changes in treatment.

Integrating Home Monitoring with Lifestyle Changes

Diet and Blood Pressure

- **Dietary Impact:** Use readings to assess how dietary choices affect your blood pressure.
- **Recipe Adjustments:** Incorporate low-sodium, heart-healthy recipes from this cookbook to improve readings.

Physical Activity

- **Exercise Effects:** Monitor how different types and intensities of exercise influence your blood pressure.

- **Stress Management:** Observe the impact of stress-reducing activities on your readings.

Tips for Success

- **Educate Yourself:** Understand what your readings mean and the factors that influence them.

- **Stay Consistent:** Regular monitoring provides the most useful data.

- **Involve Family Members:** Encourage others to monitor their blood pressure, fostering a supportive environment.

- **Device Maintenance:** Keep your monitor calibrated and replace batteries as needed.

Addressing Potential Challenges

Anxiety About Readings

- **Stay Calm:** Remember that one high reading isn't necessarily cause for alarm.

- **Focus on Trends:** Look at overall patterns rather than isolated numbers.

Technical Difficulties

- **Refer to the Manual:** Consult the device instructions for troubleshooting.

- **Customer Support:** Contact the manufacturer if issues persist.

Chapter 6: 13-Week Meal Plan

Week 1

Day 1
- **Breakfast:** Avocado and Egg Toast (p.25)
- **Lunch:** Artichoke and White Bean Salad (p.35)
- **Snack:** Stuffed Mini Peppers (p.60)
- **Dinner:** Arugula and Parmesan Salad (p.47)

Day 2
- **Breakfast:** Banana Oat Pancakes (p.25)
- **Lunch:** Balsamic Chicken and Veggie Skewers (p.35)
- **Snack:** Cucumber Avocado Bites (p.60)
- **Dinner:** Baked Cod with Lemon (p.48)

Day 3
- **Breakfast:** Berry Yogurt Parfait (p.26)
- **Lunch:** Chickpea and Spinach Stew (p.36)
- **Snack:** Garlic Parmesan Zucchini Chips (p.61)
- **Dinner:** Broccoli and Feta Pasta (p.48)

Day 4
- **Breakfast:** Caprese Avocado Toast (p.26)
- **Lunch:** Cucumber and Feta Salad (p.36)
- **Snack:** Greek Salad Skewers (p.61)
- **Dinner:** Cauliflower Rice Stir-Fry (p.49)

Day 5
- **Breakfast:** Chia Seed Pudding (p.27)
- **Lunch:** Eggplant and Tomato Stack (p.37)
- **Snack:** Hummus Stuffed Cherry Tomatoes (p.62)
- **Dinner:** Chicken and Asparagus Stir-Fry (p.49)

Day 6
- **Breakfast:** Cinnamon Apple Oatmeal (p.27)
- **Lunch:** Farro and Veggie Bowl (p.37)
- **Snack:** Mediterranean Deviled Eggs (p.62)
- **Dinner:** Chicken and Broccoli Alfredo (p.50)

Day 7
- **Breakfast:** Cottage Cheese and Fruit Bowl (p.28)
- **Lunch:** Garbanzo Bean Salad (p.38)
- **Snack:** Pesto Stuffed Mushrooms (p.63)
- **Dinner:** Chicken and Zucchini Skewers (p.50)

Week 2

Day 8
- **Breakfast:** Egg and Spinach Wrap (p.28)
- **Lunch:** Grilled Lemon Herb Chicken (p.38)
- **Snack:** Roasted Chickpeas (p.63)
- **Dinner:** Chicken Caprese (p.51)

Day 9
- **Breakfast:** Feta and Tomato Omelette (p.29)
- **Lunch:** Hummus and Veggie Wrap (p.39)
- **Snack:** Spinach and Feta Stuffed Mushrooms (p.64)
- **Dinner:** Chicken Pesto Pasta (p.51)

Day 10
- **Breakfast:** Greek Yogurt with Honey and Nuts (p.29)
- **Lunch:** Italian Tuna Salad (p.39)
- **Snack:** Tomato Basil Skewers (p.64)
- **Dinner:** Garlic Shrimp and Broccoli (p.52)

Day 11
- **Breakfast:** Mediterranean Breakfast Burrito (p.30)
- **Lunch:** Kale and Quinoa Salad (p.40)
- **Snack:** Apple Walnut Salad (p.65)
- **Dinner:** Grilled Chicken with Avocado Salsa (p.52)

Day 12
- **Breakfast:** Mushroom and Feta Scramble (p.30)
- **Lunch:** Lemon Garlic Shrimp (p.40)
- **Snack:** Beet and Goat Cheese Salad (p.65)
- **Dinner:** Grilled Eggplant with Feta (p.53)

Day 13
- **Breakfast:** Olive and Herb Frittata (p.31)
- **Lunch:** Mediterranean Chickpea Salad (p.41)
- **Snack:** Carrot and Chickpea Salad (p.66)
- **Dinner:** Lemon Herb Salmon (p.53)

Day 14
- **Breakfast:** Quinoa Breakfast Bowl (p.31)
- **Lunch:** Orzo and Spinach Salad (p.41)
- **Snack:** Citrus Avocado Salad (p.66)
- **Dinner:** Lentil and Veggie Stew (p.54)

Week 3

Day 15
- **Breakfast:** Smoked Salmon Bagel (p.32)
- **Lunch:** Pesto Zucchini Noodles (p.42)
- **Snack:** Fennel and Orange Salad (p.67)
- **Dinner:** Mediterranean Chicken Wrap (p.54)

Day 16
- **Breakfast:** Spinach and Feta Muffins (p.32)
- **Lunch:** Quinoa and Black Bean Salad (p.42)
- **Snack:** Green Bean Almondine (p.67)
- **Dinner:** Mediterranean Quinoa Bowl (p.55)

Day 17
- **Breakfast:** Tomato Basil Bruschetta (p.33)
- **Lunch:** Roasted Red Pepper Hummus Wrap (p.42)
- **Snack:** Lemon Dill Cucumber Salad (p.68)
- **Dinner:** Pasta Primavera (p.55)

Day 18
- **Breakfast:** Veggie and Hummus Wrap (p.33)
- **Lunch:** Spinach and Feta Stuffed Peppers (p.43)
- **Snack:** Peach and Arugula Salad (p.68)
- **Dinner:** Roasted Brussels Sprouts with Balsamic Glaze (p.56)

Day 19
- **Breakfast:** Yogurt and Granola Bowl (p.34)
- **Lunch:** Tomato and Cucumber Salad (p.44)
- **Snack:** Radish and Cucumber Salad (p.69)
- **Dinner:** Roasted Cauliflower Tacos (p.56)

Day 20
- **Breakfast:** Zucchini and Egg Muffins (p.34)
- **Lunch:** Tuna and White Bean Salad (p.44)
- **Snack:** Watermelon Feta Salad (p.69)
- **Dinner:** Shrimp and Avocado Salad (p.57)

Day 21
- **Breakfast:** Avocado and Egg Toast (p.25)
- **Lunch:** Veggie and Feta Stuffed Pita (p.45)
- **Snack:** Almond Butter Cookies (p.70)
- **Dinner:** Spinach and Mushroom Quesadilla (p.57)

Week 4

Day 22
- **Breakfast:** Banana Oat Pancakes (p.25)
- **Lunch:** White Bean and Kale Soup (p.45)
- **Snack:** Apple Cinnamon Bites (p.70)
- **Dinner:** Stuffed Bell Peppers (p.58)

Day 23
- **Breakfast:** Berry Yogurt Parfait (p.26)
- **Lunch:** Zesty Lemon Chicken (p.46)
- **Snack:** Berry Chia Pudding (p.71)
- **Dinner:** Tomato Basil Chicken (p.58)

Day 24
- **Breakfast:** Caprese Avocado Toast (p.26)
- **Lunch:** Zucchini and Tomato Bake (p.46)
- **Snack:** Chocolate Avocado Mousse (p.71)
- **Dinner:** Turkey and Spinach Meatballs (p.59)

Day 25
- **Breakfast:** Chia Seed Pudding (p.27)
- **Lunch:** Zucchini Noodles with Pesto (p.47)
- **Snack:** Coconut Macaroons (p.72)
- **Dinner:** Zucchini and Tomato Gratin (p.59)

Day 26
- **Breakfast:** Cinnamon Apple Oatmeal (p.27)
- **Lunch:** Artichoke and White Bean Salad (p.35)
- **Snack:** Greek Yogurt Bark (p.72)
- **Dinner:** Arugula and Parmesan Salad (p.47)

Day 27
- **Breakfast:** Cottage Cheese and Fruit Bowl (p.28)
- **Lunch:** Balsamic Chicken and Veggie Skewers (p.35)
- **Snack:** Lemon Ricotta Cheesecake (p.73)
- **Dinner:** Baked Cod with Lemon (p.48)

Day 28
- **Breakfast:** Egg and Spinach Wrap (p.28)
- **Lunch:** Chickpea and Spinach Stew (p.36)
- **Snack:** Peach Yogurt Pops (p.73)
- **Dinner:** Broccoli and Feta Pasta (p.48)

Week 5

Day 29

- **Breakfast:** Feta and Tomato Omelette (p.29)
- **Lunch:** Cucumber and Feta Salad (p.36)
- **Snack:** Strawberry Banana Smoothie Bowl (p.74)
- **Dinner:** Cauliflower Rice Stir-Fry (p.49)

Day 30

- **Breakfast:** Greek Yogurt with Honey and Nuts (p.29)
- **Lunch:** Eggplant and Tomato Stack (p.37)
- **Snack:** Vanilla Panna Cotta (p.74)
- **Dinner:** Chicken and Asparagus Stir-Fry (p.49)

Day 31

- **Breakfast:** Mediterranean Breakfast Burrito (p.30)
- **Lunch:** Farro and Veggie Bowl (p.37)
- **Snack:** Stuffed Mini Peppers (p.60)
- **Dinner:** Chicken and Broccoli Alfredo (p.50)

Day 32

- **Breakfast:** Mushroom and Feta Scramble (p.30)
- **Lunch:** Garbanzo Bean Salad (p.38)
- **Snack:** Cucumber Avocado Bites (p.60)
- **Dinner:** Chicken and Zucchini Skewers (p.50)

Day 33

- **Breakfast:** Olive and Herb Frittata (p.31)
- **Lunch:** Grilled Lemon Herb Chicken (p.38)
- **Snack:** Garlic Parmesan Zucchini Chips (p.61)
- **Dinner:** Chicken Caprese (p.51)

Day 34

- **Breakfast:** Quinoa Breakfast Bowl (p.31)
- **Lunch:** Hummus and Veggie Wrap (p.39)
- **Snack:** Greek Salad Skewers (p.61)
- **Dinner:** Chicken Pesto Pasta (p.51)

Day 35

- **Breakfast:** Smoked Salmon Bagel (p.32)
- **Lunch:** Italian Tuna Salad (p.39)
- **Snack:** Hummus Stuffed Cherry Tomatoes (p.62)
- **Dinner:** Garlic Shrimp and Broccoli (p.52)

Week 6

Day 36
- **Breakfast:** Spinach and Feta Muffins (p.32)
- **Lunch:** Kale and Quinoa Salad (p.40)
- **Snack:** Mediterranean Deviled Eggs (p.62)
- **Dinner:** Grilled Chicken with Avocado Salsa (p.52)

Day 37
- **Breakfast:** Tomato Basil Bruschetta (p.33)
- **Lunch:** Lemon Garlic Shrimp (p.40)
- **Snack:** Pesto Stuffed Mushrooms (p.63)
- **Dinner:** Grilled Eggplant with Feta (p.53)

Day 38
- **Breakfast:** Veggie and Hummus Wrap (p.33)
- **Lunch:** Mediterranean Chickpea Salad (p.41)
- **Snack:** Roasted Chickpeas (p.63)
- **Dinner:** Lemon Herb Salmon (p.53)

Day 39
- **Breakfast:** Yogurt and Granola Bowl (p.34)
- **Lunch:** Orzo and Spinach Salad (p.41)
- **Snack:** Spinach and Feta Stuffed Mushrooms (p.64)
- **Dinner:** Lentil and Veggie Stew (p.54)

Day 40
- **Breakfast:** Zucchini and Egg Muffins (p.34)
- **Lunch:** Pesto Zucchini Noodles (p.42)
- **Snack:** Tomato Basil Skewers (p.64)
- **Dinner:** Mediterranean Chicken Wrap (p.54)

Day 41
- **Breakfast:** Avocado and Egg Toast (p.25)
- **Lunch:** Quinoa and Black Bean Salad (p.42)
- **Snack:** Apple Walnut Salad (p.65)
- **Dinner:** Mediterranean Quinoa Bowl (p.55)

Day 42
- **Breakfast:** Banana Oat Pancakes (p.25)
- **Lunch:** Roasted Red Pepper Hummus Wrap (p.42)
- **Snack:** Beet and Goat Cheese Salad (p.65)
- **Dinner:** Pasta Primavera (p.55)

Week 7

Day 43
- **Breakfast:** Berry Yogurt Parfait (p.26)
- **Lunch:** Spinach and Feta Stuffed Peppers (p.43)
- **Snack:** Carrot and Chickpea Salad (p.66)
- **Dinner:** Roasted Brussels Sprouts with Balsamic Glaze (p.56)

Day 44
- **Breakfast:** Caprese Avocado Toast (p.26)
- **Lunch:** Tomato and Cucumber Salad (p.44)
- **Snack:** Citrus Avocado Salad (p.66)
- **Dinner:** Roasted Cauliflower Tacos (p.56)

Day 45
- **Breakfast:** Chia Seed Pudding (p.27)
- **Lunch:** Tuna and White Bean Salad (p.44)
- **Snack:** Fennel and Orange Salad (p.67)
- **Dinner:** Shrimp and Avocado Salad (p.57)

Day 46
- **Breakfast:** Cinnamon Apple Oatmeal (p.27)
- **Lunch:** Veggie and Feta Stuffed Pita (p.45)
- **Snack:** Green Bean Almondine (p.67)
- **Dinner:** Spinach and Mushroom Quesadilla (p.57)

Day 47
- **Breakfast:** Cottage Cheese and Fruit Bowl (p.28)
- **Lunch:** White Bean and Kale Soup (p.45)
- **Snack:** Lemon Dill Cucumber Salad (p.68)
- **Dinner:** Stuffed Bell Peppers (p.58)

Day 48
- **Breakfast:** Egg and Spinach Wrap (p.28)
- **Lunch:** Zesty Lemon Chicken (p.46)
- **Snack:** Peach and Arugula Salad (p.68)
- **Dinner:** Tomato Basil Chicken (p.58)

Day 49
- **Breakfast:** Feta and Tomato Omelette (p.29)
- **Lunch:** Zucchini and Tomato Bake (p.46)
- **Snack:** Radish and Cucumber Salad (p.69)
- **Dinner:** Turkey and Spinach Meatballs (p.59)

Week 8

Day 50

- **Breakfast:** Greek Yogurt with Honey and Nuts (p.29)
- **Lunch:** Zucchini Noodles with Pesto (p.47)
- **Snack:** Watermelon Feta Salad (p.69)
- **Dinner:** Zucchini and Tomato Gratin (p.59)

Day 51

- **Breakfast:** Mediterranean Breakfast Burrito (p.30)
- **Lunch:** Artichoke and White Bean Salad (p.35)
- **Snack:** Almond Butter Cookies (p.70)
- **Dinner:** Arugula and Parmesan Salad (p.47)

Day 52

- **Breakfast:** Mushroom and Feta Scramble (p.30)
- **Lunch:** Balsamic Chicken and Veggie Skewers (p.35)
- **Snack:** Apple Cinnamon Bites (p.70)
- **Dinner:** Baked Cod with Lemon (p.48)

Day 53

- **Breakfast:** Olive and Herb Frittata (p.31)
- **Lunch:** Chickpea and Spinach Stew (p.36)
- **Snack:** Berry Chia Pudding (p.71)
- **Dinner:** Broccoli and Feta Pasta (p.48)

Day 54

- **Breakfast:** Quinoa Breakfast Bowl (p.31)
- **Lunch:** Cucumber and Feta Salad (p.36)
- **Snack:** Chocolate Avocado Mousse (p.71)
- **Dinner:** Cauliflower Rice Stir-Fry (p.49)

Day 55

- **Breakfast:** Smoked Salmon Bagel (p.32)
- **Lunch:** Eggplant and Tomato Stack (p.37)
- **Snack:** Coconut Macaroons (p.72)
- **Dinner:** Chicken and Asparagus Stir-Fry (p.49)

Day 56

- **Breakfast:** Spinach and Feta Muffins (p.32)
- **Lunch:** Farro and Veggie Bowl (p.37)
- **Snack:** Greek Yogurt Bark (p.72)
- **Dinner:** Chicken and Broccoli Alfredo (p.50)

Week 9

Day 57
- **Breakfast:** Tomato Basil Bruschetta (p.33)
- **Lunch:** Garbanzo Bean Salad (p.38)
- **Snack:** Lemon Ricotta Cheesecake (p.73)
- **Dinner:** Chicken and Zucchini Skewers (p.50)

Day 58
- **Breakfast:** Veggie and Hummus Wrap (p.33)
- **Lunch:** Grilled Lemon Herb Chicken (p.38)
- **Snack:** Peach Yogurt Pops (p.73)
- **Dinner:** Chicken Caprese (p.51)

Day 59
- **Breakfast:** Yogurt and Granola Bowl (p.34)
- **Lunch:** Hummus and Veggie Wrap (p.39)
- **Snack:** Strawberry Banana Smoothie Bowl (p.74)
- **Dinner:** Chicken Pesto Pasta (p.51)

Day 60
- **Breakfast:** Zucchini and Egg Muffins (p.34)
- **Lunch:** Italian Tuna Salad (p.39)
- **Snack:** Vanilla Panna Cotta (p.74)
- **Dinner:** Garlic Shrimp and Broccoli (p.52)

Day 61
- **Breakfast:** Avocado and Egg Toast (p.25)
- **Lunch:** Kale and Quinoa Salad (p.40)
- **Snack:** Stuffed Mini Peppers (p.60)
- **Dinner:** Grilled Chicken with Avocado Salsa (p.52)

Day 62
- **Breakfast:** Banana Oat Pancakes (p.25)
- **Lunch:** Lemon Garlic Shrimp (p.40)
- **Snack:** Cucumber Avocado Bites (p.60)
- **Dinner:** Grilled Eggplant with Feta (p.53)

Day 63
- **Breakfast:** Berry Yogurt Parfait (p.26)
- **Lunch:** Mediterranean Chickpea Salad (p.41)
- **Snack:** Garlic Parmesan Zucchini Chips (p.61)
- **Dinner:** Lemon Herb Salmon (p.53)

Week 10

Day 64
- **Breakfast:** Caprese Avocado Toast (p.26)
- **Lunch:** Orzo and Spinach Salad (p.41)
- **Snack:** Greek Salad Skewers (p.61)
- **Dinner:** Lentil and Veggie Stew (p.54)

Day 65
- **Breakfast:** Chia Seed Pudding (p.27)
- **Lunch:** Pesto Zucchini Noodles (p.42)
- **Snack:** Hummus Stuffed Cherry Tomatoes (p.62)
- **Dinner:** Mediterranean Chicken Wrap (p.54)

Day 66
- **Breakfast:** Cinnamon Apple Oatmeal (p.27)
- **Lunch:** Quinoa and Black Bean Salad (p.42)
- **Snack:** Mediterranean Deviled Eggs (p.62)
- **Dinner:** Mediterranean Quinoa Bowl (p.55)

Day 67
- **Breakfast:** Cottage Cheese and Fruit Bowl (p.28)
- **Lunch:** Roasted Red Pepper Hummus Wrap (p.42)
- **Snack:** Pesto Stuffed Mushrooms (p.63)
- **Dinner:** Pasta Primavera (p.55)

Day 68
- **Breakfast:** Egg and Spinach Wrap (p.28)
- **Lunch:** Spinach and Feta Stuffed Peppers (p.43)
- **Snack:** Roasted Chickpeas (p.63)
- **Dinner:** Roasted Brussels Sprouts with Balsamic Glaze (p.56)

Day 69
- **Breakfast:** Feta and Tomato Omelette (p.29)
- **Lunch:** Tomato and Cucumber Salad (p.44)
- **Snack:** Spinach and Feta Stuffed Mushrooms (p.64)
- **Dinner:** Roasted Cauliflower Tacos (p.56)

Day 70
- **Breakfast:** Greek Yogurt with Honey and Nuts (p.29)
- **Lunch:** Tuna and White Bean Salad (p.44)
- **Snack:** Tomato Basil Skewers (p.64)
- **Dinner:** Shrimp and Avocado Salad (p.57)

Week 11

Day 71
- **Breakfast:** Mediterranean Breakfast Burrito (p.30)
- **Lunch:** Veggie and Feta Stuffed Pita (p.45)
- **Snack:** Apple Walnut Salad (p.65)
- **Dinner:** Spinach and Mushroom Quesadilla (p.57)

Day 72
- **Breakfast:** Mushroom and Feta Scramble (p.30)
- **Lunch:** White Bean and Kale Soup (p.45)
- **Snack:** Beet and Goat Cheese Salad (p.65)
- **Dinner:** Stuffed Bell Peppers (p.58)

Day 73
- **Breakfast:** Olive and Herb Frittata (p.31)
- **Lunch:** Zesty Lemon Chicken (p.46)
- **Snack:** Carrot and Chickpea Salad (p.66)
- **Dinner:** Tomato Basil Chicken (p.58)

Day 74
- **Breakfast:** Quinoa Breakfast Bowl (p.31)
- **Lunch:** Zucchini and Tomato Bake (p.46)
- **Snack:** Citrus Avocado Salad (p.66)
- **Dinner:** Turkey and Spinach Meatballs (p.59)

Day 75
- **Breakfast:** Smoked Salmon Bagel (p.32)
- **Lunch:** Zucchini Noodles with Pesto (p.47)
- **Snack:** Fennel and Orange Salad (p.67)
- **Dinner:** Zucchini and Tomato Gratin (p.59)

Day 76
- **Breakfast:** Spinach and Feta Muffins (p.32)
- **Lunch:** Artichoke and White Bean Salad (p.35)
- **Snack:** Green Bean Almondine (p.67)
- **Dinner:** Arugula and Parmesan Salad (p.47)

Day 77
- **Breakfast:** Tomato Basil Bruschetta (p.33)
- **Lunch:** Balsamic Chicken and Veggie Skewers (p.35)
- **Snack:** Lemon Dill Cucumber Salad (p.68)
- **Dinner:** Baked Cod with Lemon (p.48)

Week 12

Day 78

- **Breakfast:** Veggie and Hummus Wrap (p.33)
- **Lunch:** Chickpea and Spinach Stew (p.36)
- **Snack:** Peach and Arugula Salad (p.68)
- **Dinner:** Broccoli and Feta Pasta (p.48)

Day 79

- **Breakfast:** Yogurt and Granola Bowl (p.34)
- **Lunch:** Cucumber and Feta Salad (p.36)
- **Snack:** Radish and Cucumber Salad (p.69)
- **Dinner:** Cauliflower Rice Stir-Fry (p.49)

Day 80

- **Breakfast:** Zucchini and Egg Muffins (p.34)
- **Lunch:** Eggplant and Tomato Stack (p.37)
- **Snack:** Watermelon Feta Salad (p.69)
- **Dinner:** Chicken and Asparagus Stir-Fry (p.49)

Day 81

- **Breakfast:** Avocado and Egg Toast (p.25)
- **Lunch:** Farro and Veggie Bowl (p.37)
- **Snack:** Almond Butter Cookies (p.70)
- **Dinner:** Chicken and Broccoli Alfredo (p.50)

Day 82

- **Breakfast:** Banana Oat Pancakes (p.25)
- **Lunch:** Garbanzo Bean Salad (p.38)
- **Snack:** Apple Cinnamon Bites (p.70)
- **Dinner:** Chicken and Zucchini Skewers (p.50)

Day 83

- **Breakfast:** Berry Yogurt Parfait (p.26)
- **Lunch:** Grilled Lemon Herb Chicken (p.38)
- **Snack:** Berry Chia Pudding (p.71)
- **Dinner:** Chicken Caprese (p.51)

Day 84

- **Breakfast:** Caprese Avocado Toast (p.26)
- **Lunch:** Hummus and Veggie Wrap (p.39)
- **Snack:** Chocolate Avocado Mousse (p.71)
- **Dinner:** Chicken Pesto Pasta (p.51)

Week 13

Day 85
- **Breakfast:** Chia Seed Pudding (p.27)
- **Lunch:** Italian Tuna Salad (p.39)
- **Snack:** Coconut Macaroons (p.72)
- **Dinner:** Garlic Shrimp and Broccoli (p.52)

Day 86
- **Breakfast:** Cinnamon Apple Oatmeal (p.27)
- **Lunch:** Kale and Quinoa Salad (p.40)
- **Snack:** Greek Yogurt Bark (p.72)
- **Dinner:** Grilled Chicken with Avocado Salsa (p.52)

Day 87
- **Breakfast:** Cottage Cheese and Fruit Bowl (p.28)
- **Lunch:** Lemon Garlic Shrimp (p.40)
- **Snack:** Lemon Ricotta Cheesecake (p.73)
- **Dinner:** Grilled Eggplant with Feta (p.53)

Day 88
- **Breakfast:** Egg and Spinach Wrap (p.28)
- **Lunch:** Mediterranean Chickpea Salad (p.41)
- **Snack:** Peach Yogurt Pops (p.73)
- **Dinner:** Lemon Herb Salmon (p.53)

Day 89
- **Breakfast:** Feta and Tomato Omelette (p.29)
- **Lunch:** Orzo and Spinach Salad (p.41)
- **Snack:** Strawberry Banana Smoothie Bowl (p.74)
- **Dinner:** Lentil and Veggie Stew (p.54)

Day 90
- **Breakfast:** Greek Yogurt with Honey and Nuts (p.29)
- **Lunch:** Pesto Zucchini Noodles (p.42)
- **Snack:** Vanilla Panna Cotta (p.74)
- **Dinner:** Mediterranean Chicken Wrap (p.54)

Conclusion

Embarking on the journey of the 5-Ingredient Mediterranean DASH Diet Cookbook, readers have been equipped with a comprehensive guide that merges the heart-healthy Mediterranean diet with the blood pressure-lowering DASH diet. This fusion creates a powerful dietary approach that not only aims at improving cardiovascular health but also at managing weight effectively, all while ensuring the meals remain simple, delicious, and quick to prepare.

The essence of this cookbook lies in its simplicity and the profound impact it can have on one's health. By focusing on whole, nutrient-rich foods and limiting processed and high-sodium options, individuals can naturally steer their health towards a better path. The recipes provided, all requiring no more than five ingredients, demonstrate that eating healthily does not have to be complicated or time-consuming.

Moreover, the inclusion of a budget-friendly weekly shopping list and a guide to reading and understanding food labels empowers readers to make informed choices beyond the recipes in this book. It's about adopting a lifestyle that values quality over quantity, flavor over blandness, and health over convenience.

As readers continue to explore and experiment with the recipes and tips provided, they'll find that managing blood pressure, losing weight, and improving heart health can be achieved not just through medication but also through enjoyable dietary changes. This book serves as a testament to the power of combining two scientifically backed diets and simplifying them for everyday use, making it an invaluable resource for anyone looking to embrace a healthier lifestyle without sacrificing taste or their budget.

Conversion Charts

Length

US (inches)	UK (centimeters)
1 inch	2.54 cm
12 inches (1 foot)	30.48 cm

Volume

US	UK Equivalent
1 teaspoon	4.93 ml
1 tablespoon	14.79 ml
1 fluid ounce	29.57 ml
1 cup	236.59 ml
1 pint (16 fl oz)	473.18 ml
1 quart (32 fl oz)	946.35 ml
1 gallon (128 fl oz)	3.785 L

Weight

US	UK Equivalent
1 ounce	28.35 grams
1 pound	453.59 grams
1 stone	6.35 kg

Cooking Temperature

Fahrenheit (°F)	Celsius (°C)
32°F (freezing point of water)	0°C
212°F (boiling point of water)	100°C
250°F	120°C
275°F	135°C
300°F	150°C
325°F	160°C
350°F	175°C
375°F	190°C
400°F	200°C
425°F	220°C
450°F	230°C
475°F	245°C

Thank you so much for purchasing my book! I'm thrilled to have you as part of my reading family.

If you could take a moment to scan the QR code below and leave your honest review on Amazon, I would be deeply grateful.

If you are reading the ebook version, please click on this link:

https://www.amazon.com/review/create-review?&ASIN=B0DJC2P7W5

Your feedback is incredibly important to me—it helps me grow as a writer and makes our community stronger. I genuinely love hearing from you and value your thoughts immensely!

Made in United States
Troutdale, OR
01/07/2025

27698886R00060